An Insider's Guide to

Getting the Best
out of the Health System

Kate Ryder

MPH, BA(Hons), RN

This is an IndieMosh book

brought to you by MoshPit Publishing
an imprint of Mosher's Business Support Pty Ltd

PO BOX 147
Hazelbrook NSW 2779

www.indiemosh.com.au

Cataloguing-in-Publication entry is available from the National
Library of Australia: http://catalogue.nla.gov.au/

Title: An insider's guide to getting the best out of the health
             system

Author: Ryder, Kate

ISBNs: 978-1-925353-30-3 (paperback)
             978-1-925353-31-0 (ebook – epub)
             978-1-925353-32-7 (ebook – mobi)

Cover design by Ally Mosher, IndieMosh
Cover images: *Patient Space* and *Treatment* © Kate Ryder 2014
Illustrations by Liz Mackie wormsey15@gmail.com
Author's photograph by Alexis Bartlett alexis@peapodphoto.com

Dedications

This book is dedicated to my late mother, Beryl Ryder, late father, Ron Ryder and late friend Karen Williams who discharged herself from a hospital as a terminally ill patient while uttering the immortal words: "This hospital is detrimental to my health". You have all inspired me to write this book.

To my old dog, Billie, who was beside me while I wrote this book and who died on the eve of its publication.

Lastly, to my partner Jane Wilson, who supported and encouraged me throughout the process and who thankfully is still very much alive.

A heart-felt thank you to you all.

About the author

Kate Ryder is a registered nurse with more than 20 years of clinical experience in both public and private hospitals in England and here in Australia, and in a range of different specialities. These range from emergency, intensive care, general medical, surgical and short-stay wards, oncology, rehabilitation, palliative care, occupational health and community nursing.

Kate has also worked as a patient support officer and as a senior investigator with the Office of the Health Care Complaints Commission. At the Commission she investigated complaints which led to the de-registration of a number of registered health professionals, and the amendment and formulation of a number of hospital and State Government health policies and procedures. During her 10 years at the Commission, she also contributed to the establishment of the Patient Support Office, wrote case-histories for the Commission's annual reports and the Commission's Health Investigator journal, and addressed a number of community groups and gave media interviews about the work of the Patient Support Office and the Commission.

While working as a nurse, Kate conducted a quantitative and qualitative research study into the reasons why patients leave the emergency department without being seen by a doctor. She undertook this research in the emergency department of St. Vincent's Public Hospital, Darlinghurst in 1996, as part of a Masters of Public Health (MPH) course at the University of New South Wales. This research later informed the Office of the Health Care Complaints Commission's position on the treatment of the mentally ill in emergency departments, which in part led to the establishment of Psychiatric Emergency Care Centres (PECC) units in emergency departments in New South Wales.

More recently, Kate has been working casually as a registered nurse while also working as an advocate.

She assisted the parents of a young Malay Chinese man whose death was the subject of a coronial investigation by the NSW Coroner's Office.

The young man died in an acute psychiatric ward from acute bronchial pneumonia, secondary to multi-drug toxicity. The only drugs in his body were those prescribed by his treating doctors and administered by the nurses looking after him on the ward.

In what appears to be an Australian if not a world first, his post-mortem blood was used for pharmacogenomic testing, the results of which were considered by the Coroner when establishing the cause of death.

Preface

The decisions and choices we make as patients are often based on assumptions such as: doctors are saints and nurses are angels; everyone has my best interests at heart; everyone knows what they are doing and are doing it to the best of their ability, properly and safely; someone will tell me when things are going wrong; and hospitals are safe places to be. If I can achieve just two things with this book it will be these:

- To convince you that you cannot make such assumptions.

- To encourage you to take a more active role in protecting yourself and others as patients.

I knew this was a book that needed to be written when a colleague remarked: "You haven't told them that have you?", after I informed her I had written in this book that no intravenous antibiotic should be administered to a patient in less than two to three minutes because of the damage it may do to a patient's vein. As you can see, some of my professional colleagues are seemingly concerned with patients knowing what should happen to them in hospital. This book is written with you and with them in mind.

While for the most part health professionals are taught what they need to know to look after patients, they are generally not taught how to teach patients to look after themselves, or even what to teach them. This is often done on an individual and ad-hoc basis if it is done at all.

It is the patient who has always been missing from discussions when governments try to reform or improve the health system. It is my contention that, if you can educate the patient as to what should happen to them in hospital and how to protect themselves as patients, you can greatly reduce the risks of mistakes or adverse events occurring to them and to others in the future.

In saying this, however, just knowing what should happen and what you can do about it is not enough. You have to act on what you see and hear happening to you and to others as patients, however uncomfortable this may be for you at the time. Unfortunately, this will probably be at a time when you are most vulnerable and when you are least able to do so – when you are a patient. This will remain a challenge.

As the title of the book implies, this book is intended as a guide only. Hospital, medical and nursing practices vary from specialist to specialist, from speciality to speciality, from ward to ward, from hospital to hospital, and from health authority to health authority.

I have tried to include all the things most patients need to know, and specific details of how to care for yourself when undergoing certain procedures. An example of this is the insertion of a urinary catheter, which most patients will not undergo.

This book is applicable to all Western style health services in both the public and private sector.

For the ease of writing I will refer to all doctors as being 'she' instead of she/he, unless I am referring to someone in particular.

Finally, I would like to take the opportunity to thank all those who have helped me in the writing of this book. Firstly, I would like to thank those who offered advice, support, suggestions and wise counsel on the content of the book. This includes Jane

Wilson, Dr. Joanne Morgan, Liz Rehfeldt, Liz Mackie, Nancy Rehfeldt, and my nursing colleagues who are too many to mention individually.

Secondly I would like to thank Liz Mackie for her entertaining and insightful illustrations and Alexis Bartlett for my Author's photograph.

Thirdly, I would like to thank Liz Rehfeldt again for the initial editing of the text, Lyn Fletcher for additional editing, proof reading and stylistic recommendations for the text, and MoshPit Publishing for publishing this text.

Lastly, I would like to thank Jane Wilson again and Christine Bain for all the 'support services' they provided while I wrote this text. It was a real team effort, thank you.

Kate Ryder
Sydney, Australia, 2015

Contents

WHAT YOU NEED TO KNOW ON ADMISSION TO HOSPITAL 65

Chapter 1:
Before you go to hospital

TIME TO ACT

You can become very sick, very quickly at times, sometimes to the extent that you cannot even communicate. Consequently, it is important to always:

- find out how to call an ambulance in the country where you are living or staying

- keep two copies of an up-to-date printed record of your medical history and your current medication

- know where your nearest hospital emergency department is.

Keeping a written record of your medical history and medication

Your personalised medical record needs to be readily available for any locum general practitioner (GP) who treats you at home and is unfamiliar with your medical history, and for any ambulance officer who arrives to take you to hospital. Keep it in a place where it can be easily seen and label the outside of the folder in which it is kept so it is easily identifiable. Ideally you should also keep a spare copy with your next-of-kin or entrusted friend. This is especially important if you:

- have difficulty communicating verbally

- are becoming forgetful in any way

- are from a culturally and linguistically diverse (CaLD) background
- have an intellectual disability
- have a complicated medical history
- have life-threatening and medically authenticated allergies
- are on a number of different medications
- intend travelling overseas
- may have been the victim of identity fraud.

Ideally, your medical record should also contain copies of the reports of any investigations and electrocardiographs (ECGs) you have had done in the past, and copies of any legal documents you may have such as your 'Enduring Power of Attorney' or 'End of Life Directive'. You can ask any technician who performs an ECG on you if you can have a copy for your medical file. Most ECG machines can print an additional copy.

If you arrive with a complete copy of your medical record you will generally be assessed more quickly and efficiently and your treatment potentially started sooner.

Your medical record should include a record of the following:

My medical record

- treating GP(s) and their current contact details

- name and contact details of current specialist(s)

- Medicare number and Private Health Insurance details (if applicable)

- next-of-kin, 'Enduring Power of Attorney' and/or patient advocate and their contact details

- past and current medical illnesses, previous operations and details of where and when these occurred

- any medical investigations you have had to date, where these were conducted and when

- current medications and alternative medications

- any allergies, side-effects, or adverse events you have experienced to any medications, skin dressings, anaesthetic drugs, foods or intravenous contrast mediums

- childhood illnesses and vaccinations

- height and weight

- blood group if you know it

- results of any genetic testing if you have had this done

- pharmacogenomic profile if you have had this done (more about this in the section on 'Protecting yourself').

For CaLD background patients this medical file should:

- be written in your own language and in English if possible

- include details of your country and region of birth, and the language(s) and dialect(s) you speak

- include the contact details of someone who can speak English on your behalf if possible (including their work, home and mobile phone numbers, and details of your relationship with them)

- include written authorisation for this nominated person to speak and receive information about you, and on your behalf.

As a back-up, and especially if you have life-threatening allergies or medical conditions such as epilepsy or diabetes which can render you confused or even unconscious at times, you might want to join a not-for-profit organisation such as MedicAlert.

MedicAlert is an online Australian organisation that offers 24-hour a day emergency medical access to your stored health information and an identification service.

You indicate your annual membership of such an organisation by wearing an easily identifiable bracelet or necklace on which is printed the MedicAlert logo. For more information, visit their website on www.medicalert.org.au.

So you think something might be wrong with you

The first thing most people experience as a potential patient is that they think or know something is wrong with them. This can occur suddenly and 'out-of-the-blue' or it can occur slowly over days, weeks, months or even years.

Where pain is involved, the symptoms you experience can vary. They can range from such things as:

- a vague feeling of discomfort or persistent fullness in the abdomen

- to a nagging pain in a shoulder

- to the sensation akin to that of an elephant sitting on your chest.

The intensity of these symptoms will generally govern what you should do about it. As a general rule, if you ignore or delay doing something about these symptoms, and there is something seriously wrong with you, you will almost certainly diminish your chances of recovering from or even surviving it.

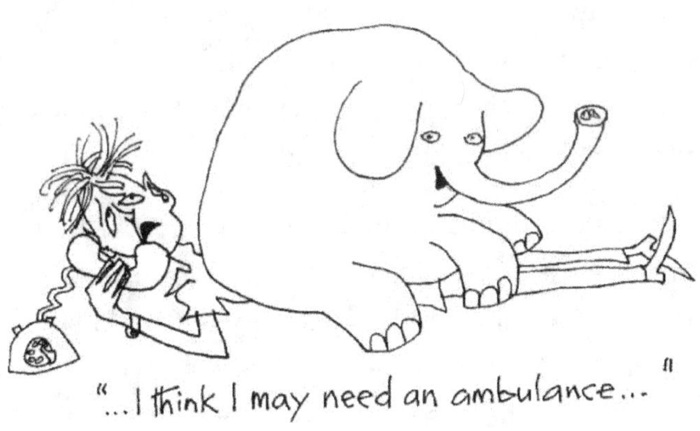

THIS IS A CRUCIAL MOMENT in the life of any potential patient and it is to you or your friends or relatives that this book is directed. To those of you who choose to ignore or to delay seeking treatment, or to involve yourself in inadequate or incomplete treatment, this book will probably not help you.

Call an ambulance or see a general practitioner?

The major advice I would give if you are considering whether to call an ambulance or not is this: if you think you are ill enough to consider calling for an ambulance, call one. Any social embarrassment you may feel if there is little wrong with you should have no place in caring for your health or the health of others.

If you call an ambulance and you are not very ill, the worst that will happen is that you will have a long wait in the emergency department, you will have to pay for the ambulance, and you may feel a little bit silly. This is a small price for saving one's life.

Do not leave the decision making or action to others

For those of you who have friends or relatives suffering with a medical condition, do not assume any advice you have given will be heeded or followed. Do not think it will be heeded even if they know you are a health professional. Any proposed action is best initiated by you if at all possible.

This was sadly brought home to me in 2006, when over the phone from Australia I asked my then 86-year-old father in England to ring for an ambulance for my mother. I stressed how important it was for him to do this straight away. He gave me the impression that he understood the importance of what I was saying and more importantly would act on my advice. I was wrong, and sadly it cost my mother the remaining years of her life.

Not wanting to offend their locum GP who had visited the day before and had failed to adequately treat my mother's overloaded bowel, and not wanting to 'make a fuss' as was his

Always call an ambulance if you or anyone has:

- difficulty breathing, is choking, or is making an odd sound when they breathe

- any kind of chest pain or tightness, severe abdominal pain, or sudden, intense headache

- severe burns in adults or any burns in young children

- had a sudden collapse or unexplained fall

- swallowed any household chemicals

- been electrocuted or involved in a motor vehicle accident or an industrial accident where the person has been injured or trapped, or fallen from a height

- sustained any penetrating injury to the body (do not try to remove the object)

- unexplained fitting or seizures or infants that are fitting or have an ongoing fever

- any kind of bleeding that will not stop or you don't know if it has stopped

- been unconscious for any length of time or has a decreased level of consciousness

- any kind of facial drooping, difficulty speaking or any kind of weakness in your body

- inhaled any kind of smoke or water, or has nearly drowned

- attempted suicide.

nature, my late father, Ron did not call for an ambulance. Instead he called their GP's locum service again.

By the time the doctor arrived for the second time over two hours later, it was too late. My mother's bowel had perforated at home or on her way to hospital, and she later died in hospital.

To this day I deeply regret not having called the ambulance myself from Australia, and my father came to deeply regret his decision not to call the ambulance when asked to do so too. Please learn from our mistakes and don't ignore your 'Ron Ring' moment.

Let your doctor diagnose your medical condition

Looking up your symptoms on the internet or telling your wife or friend about the condition that ails you, and having them decide if you should seek advice or treatment for the condition, is, as you can imagine, a poor substitute for going to your local doctor and telling her yourself. Self-explanatory you would think, but if I had a dollar for every patient who has told me they had asked their wife or a friend if they should seek treatment or advice I would be fully retired by now.

And, just because you have the same signs and symptoms as someone else does not mean you have the same problem as them. For instance, just because the blood in Joe's stool was caused by a haemorrhoid in Joe's rectum does not mean that the blood in your stool is caused by a haemorrhoid in yours.

One of the poorly recognised conditions for women is a heart attack. Given that the rate of coronary artery disease is increasing in women, which predisposes them to having more heart attacks, it is important this condition is quickly recognised by the women themselves and by health professionals.

When women have a heart attack it can present in different ways than it does in men. Whereas most men have chest pain when they are experience a heart attack, some women experience a heart attack as pain just below the rib cage. Consequently, a heart attack in women can go unrecognised as such by the women themselves and by others. In addition, women often put up with this pain in the early stages rather than seeking immediate medical care.

Remember, the quicker you do something about the medical condition that ails or troubles you the better the chance the doctor has of diagnosing your condition and stopping it from getting worse. Ultimately, it can save or at least prolong your life. IT IS AS SIMPLE AS THAT.

The importance of medication expiry dates

All medications have expiry dates. These are usually printed on the side of the medication bottle and/or box, or on the sleeve of tablets and can be very difficult to see. It is important your medications have not expired.

If you have trouble seeing the expiry date of your medication, ask the pharmacist to write it down for you. This is especially important if you use the medication infrequently such as Ventolin™, EpiPens® and glyceryl trinitrate (GTN). This is because the effectiveness of the medication starts to diminish when the medication has passed its expiry date. If necessary, put the expiry date in your diary well before it is due.

For life threatening conditions, such as asthma that requires Ventolin™ and certain allergies that require an EpiPen®, it is important you have back-up supplies and these are readily accessible at all times.

GETTING THE BEST OUT OF YOUR GENERAL PRACTITIONER

Choosing a general practitioner (GP)

General Practitioners (GPs) are the linchpins of the health system. Their primary role is to keep you well from the day you are born to the moment you die. They attempt to do this when they:

- give you your childhood vaccinations

- monitor your overall development, waist measurement and body mass index from your weight and height, with reference to national and international guidelines as to what is considered normal for your age and sex

- check the regularity and the number of your heart beats by taking your pulse with their fingers or listening to your heart with a stethoscope and check your blood pressure, at least once a year

- give you advice about healthy eating habits, the value of regular exercise, avoiding smoking and illicit drugs and limiting your intake of alcohol

- monitor your overall health by doing such things as routine observations and blood tests, by weighing you, and by doing routine screening for such things as breast cancer (breast examination), an enlarged prostate, and the papilloma virus (Pap smears)

- identify what ails you by organising such things as:

  o blood tests, x-rays and scans

  o referrals to specialists

  o monitoring your ongoing care

- attempt to prevent you from getting worse when they:

  o prescribe medications for you, advise you how these work and their possible side-effects, and monitor the effectiveness of them on you

  o refer you to a specialist skilled in treating your particular illness or condition, or have you admitted to hospital.

If your GP is not doing these types of things, consider choosing another GP.

At the very least, your GP should:

- be able to provide you with information with which you can keep yourself well

- be able to make you feel safe and comfortable in their presence by doing and saying things that enable you to feel so

- provide you with access to national health screening programs

- give you a complete medical examination when you are unwell

- be able to arrive at a provisional or actual diagnosis of your medical illness

- refer you onto a specialist if your medical illness is outside their field of expertise

At the very least, your GP should (cont.):

- be familiar with your medical illness and current methods of treating it

- be able to tell you the aim of any treatment they propose to provide for you (for instance, if the aim of treatment is to treat the condition or to prevent it from getting worse, she will be able to tell you when this has been achieved)

- monitor the effects of their treatment on you (for instance, if your GP has prescribed you blood pressure lowering medication, she should be checking to make sure this is happening).

Your GP should not:

- Perform medical procedures outside their field of expertise.

- Prescribe narcotic analgesia such as oxycodone or OxyContin® on an ongoing and regular basis without: a) obtaining an authority to do so from the health department, and b) without referring you on to a pain clinic if this is required of GPs and if these are available. This should be the case unless of course you are receiving palliative care.

Your GP should not (cont.):

- Examine your child's penis unless your child's presenting medical condition relates to his penis, he has a suspected urinary tract infection, he has problems passing urine, or he has a suspected hormone imbalance.

- Examine your child's testicles unless your child has a lump in their testicles, he has or has had mumps, he has a suspected hormone imbalance, or he is examined as a baby to see if his testicles have descended down into the scrotal sac.

- Put his finger in your child's anus unless your child is a new born baby and has not passed meconium after 48 hours, has a suspected injury in that area, is constipated, is bleeding from the anus, or is suspected of having appendicitis.

- Ask your child to masturbate in front of him.

- Examine your vagina or breasts unless this is part of an annual screening program or your presenting medical condition relates to these areas of the body, such as you have pain in your abdomen or a lump in your breast. Ask for a chaperone if you feel uncomfortable.

Your therapeutic relationship with your GP will arguably be the most important professional relationship you will have with anyone in your life. I would strongly advise you to respect and nurture this relationship as if it is with a dear friend. However, if you do not feel comfortable with your GP (or with any doctor for that matter) because they say or do things which make you feel uncomfortable, embarrassed or even afraid, and you cannot talk to or confide in your GP, consider finding another one.

If you live in a city or large town there are plenty to choose from. If you live in a regional or rural area where your choice is limited, take a trusted friend along with you to the consultations.

The importance of having a regular general practitioner

Many people do not have a regular GP or cannot nominate one they see on a regular basis. Consequently, the medical information that exists for them can be scattered among a number of different GPs in a number of different practices. Even less people have signed up for Australia's centralised electronic health system.

If your medical information is scattered among a number of GPs, then your medical history will potentially remain unknown and unavailable for access by each GP that sees you. As you can imagine, this is fraught with danger.

While it is important to have a regular general practitioner it is just as important to have a regular pharmacist. This is because your pharmacist:

- will know all the medications that have been prescribed for you
- will know which medications are likely to interact

- is more likely to make themselves available to discuss your medications with you, and

- can advise you when you should take your medications. For instance, calcium carbonate should not be taken within 4-5 hours of thyroxine.

Planning your visit to the general practitioner

When you are making an appointment to see your GP for a new or worsening medical condition, ask the practice's receptionist for a long appointment. A standard or level A (less than 5 minutes) consultation is simply not enough time for your GP to give your new or worsening medical condition the attention it requires.

Some GPs will extend the consultation time in keeping with the time required to investigate or treat your presenting medical condition, others will not. At these times you will be asked to make another appointment and come back at a later date. Worse still, the GP may not examine you as thoroughly as they should and will invariably not take a complete medical and social history from you.

For a new medical condition or the worsening of a pre-existing medical condition you will need a long appointment. This should be at least a level B (more than 5 minutes and less than 20 minutes) if not a level C (20–40 minutes) consultation.

With regard to the development of a new medical condition, make sure you write down in advance such things as:

- when the condition started, how it affects you, and when

- what, if anything makes it worse or better

- what reliable others have noticed about your condition and when

- if anyone from your extended family has, or has had, the same or similar medical condition.

The advantage of preparing for your visit in advance is that you stay focused during the consultation and you do not waste your consultation time.

If you think that, on average, people only hear about 40 percent of any conversation you have with them, it is important you only provide relevant information to the GP.

As you can imagine, it is not important for your GP to know how many cream buns you ate that day if you are not a diabetic. It is not important for her to know what your friend Marjorie thinks, if Marjorie's thoughts are unrelated to your presenting medical condition. You do not want the most important aspect of your medical story to be lost in the missing 60 percent of the conversation.

Ideally, you should take your medications with you to your consultation.

Do not forget to mention the medications you keep in the fridge, and which you should leave in the fridge when you attend the consultation.

Mention any fruit juices or supplementary or alternative medications you are also taking. Mention these to your pharmacist too. This is because some of these alternative medications can interact with the other medications prescribed for you, and your general practitioner, especially if they are inexperienced, will not necessarily know which ones will. For example, Saint John's Wort and grapefruit juice can inhibit several important cytochrome P450 enzymes.

Cytochrome P450 enzymes are necessary for the bioactivation of the chemicals in the medications so they can be used by the body, and used to breakdown the medications so they can be finally excreted from your body. More about this in the section on 'Medications can make you feel sick or have no therapeutic benefit'.

Your GP will also need to know your entire medical history. This is especially true of the medical history she is unaware of or may have forgotten about.

Do not be selective about the information you give her or think certain things are not relevant. For instance, the hernia you had repaired in your left groin could now be the cause of the pain in your right shoulder, or the bowel surgery you had could now be affecting the ability of your body to break down or metabolise the drugs that have since been prescribed for you. Take your updated medical file with you.

Your GP will also need to know if you smoke and drink and how much of these you consume. Be honest. If you drink two bottles of wine a day, say so. Your GP will not judge you. Your GP will not be shocked by your disclosure and has almost certainly heard it all before. I once looked after a barrister who regularly drank 1½ bottles of spirits a day.

Mention all of your medical conditions to your GP, even if you find it embarrassing to do so. They could be indicative of a more serious underlying problem. If you are suffering from an embarrassing medical condition, your GP will almost certainly be familiar with it. She will not think badly of you if you talk about the problem.

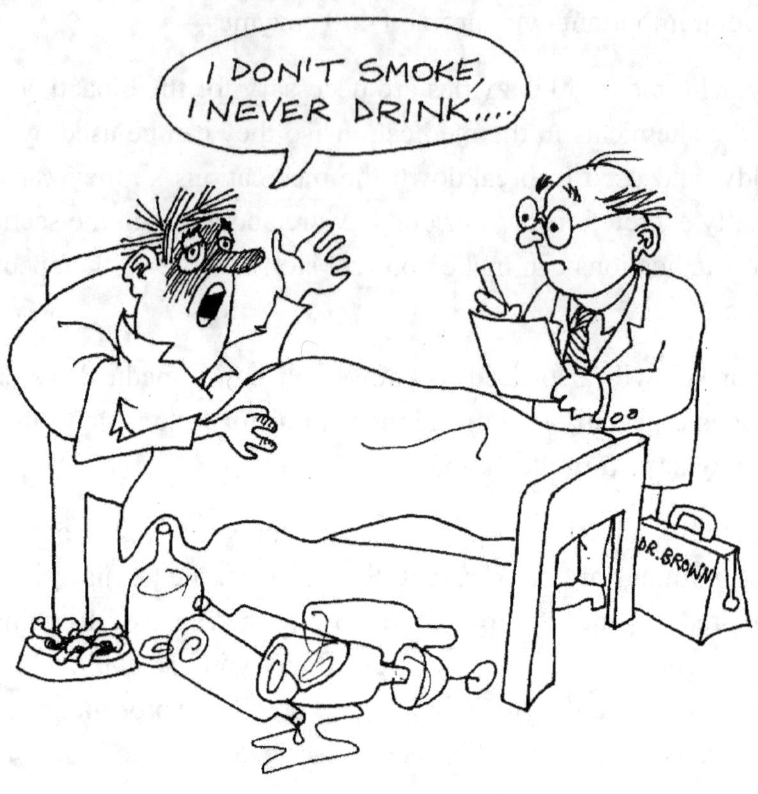

Take a quick look at www.channel4embarrassingillnesses.com to see that you are not alone, and that you share your particular problem or concern with others. Plus, if patients do not disclose details of embarrassing problems they have, medical researchers will not know the extent of these problems. They will have little incentive to try to do anything about them.

In addition to writing down the details of your medical condition in advance of your consultation, you may want to think about the things you want to ask your GP. This is especially important if she prescribes you medication for your new medical condition or organises for you to have additional tests or investigations.

Things you might want to ask your GP

- What is your experience of treating this particular condition?

- Could my medical condition be connected to the medications I am taking?

- When can I expect to feel better?

- If I don't feel better by _______, when should I come back to see you?

- If I do not take the medication you want to prescribe for me, what is likely to happen?

- What are the side-effects of these tablets and can they interact with my other tablets?

- When can I expect the results, and how can I follow up on the results if I haven't heard anything?

- Do you think I need a referral to a specialist?

- Can I have a copy of your referral letter to the specialist?

- Why have I have developed this condition?

- Does this condition run in families? (If 'Yes')

- Should my immediate and extended family have genetic counselling or testing?

Finally, in preparation for your visit to your GP's practice, wear clothes you can easily remove. Avoid wearing layers upon layers of clothes. You do not want your precious consultation time taken up with dressing and undressing.

Importance of updating your contact details

Make sure the GP's receptionist has your current contact details. If you change addresses or phone numbers at any time, make sure you update your contact details with your GP's receptionist. This is because you may need investigations in the future and you will need to be able to be contacted regarding the results.

Getting your results

Familiarise yourself with your GP's usual practice by asking the receptionist who will contact you regarding your results. If you change surgeries, do not assume that all GPs practice in the same way and that they do so all the time. Finally, do not assume that just because you haven't heard from someone that everything is fine. Ring and check. Remember, irrespective of how good or efficient people seem to be, mistakes can and do occur at times.

Looking up signs and symptoms on the internet

It is alright to look up your signs and symptoms on the internet. At times it can make you aware of other signs or symptoms you have been experiencing, and which you may not have thought were connected.

However, if you have signs or symptoms or conditions that are the same or similar to those outlined under the heading 'Call an ambulance or see a general practitioner?' do not waste time looking them up on the internet. Call an ambulance.

While looking things up on the internet can help some people, it can cause unnecessary worry for others. This is especially true for those prone to anxiety.

Protecting your relationship with your GP

If you do look up signs and symptoms on the internet and think you can identify what is wrong with you, do not make up additional symptoms you read about, or exaggerate the symptoms you have, just to 'fit' the illness you think you may have.

If you attempt to mislead your GP in this way you can be easily diagnosed with the wrong medical condition. Plus, if your GP suspects, or knows you are exaggerating or even fabricating signs and symptoms you do not have, it will almost certainly damage the professional relationship you have with her. Do not compromise this professional relationship with potentially unfounded fears and beliefs and inappropriate actions.

Some patients deliberately conceal or omit relevant information from their doctors. This has been borne out with reference to patient's old clinical notes, from enquiries made of other hospitals, and discovered during surgical operations or investigative procedures. Your professional relationship with your doctors should be based on mutual respect, co-operation and above all honesty.

Do not assume a GP is not very good because you cannot get in to see her when you want to. Do not assume your GP is not very good because she doesn't automatically remember you or your entire medical history when you do see her. If your GP is good and/or experienced, and/or works in a busy general practice, she will have a number of patients. She cannot be expected to necessarily remember everything about each and every one of them. This is especially true of patients she only sees on an ad hoc basis.

This is the time for a plug for a regular GP – I would ask you to consider these simple questions:

- Which GP is likely to:
    - take the time to get to know you as a person
    - be experienced with your unique medical history
    - be more likely to pick up on any deterioration in your general health
    - will care about you on an ongoing basis
    - will have your entire medical history to hand
    - will probably have an intimate working knowledge of your unique family and social history?

- Would you prefer a GP in a bulk billing medical centre who only works there on an intermittent or locum basis, or one in an upfront, fee paying and stable family medical practice?

Ways you can help your GP to look after you in the future

There are a number ways you can help your GP to look after you. These include:

- not delaying seeing your GP

- not buying your medications or other health related products from potentially unregulated sources online

- not taking out-of-date medications

- not seeking strong analgesia or mind altering medication from several GPs

- not sharing medications with family members

- not taking previously prescribed medications such as antibiotics for new infections

- asking your GP to prescribe generic, cheaper (but just as good) versions of the same drugs, rather than reaching the decision you cannot afford the drugs prescribed for you

- taking your medications properly and according to the directions on the packet

- talking to your doctor if your need for medication such as Ventolin™ increases, rather than simply taking more Ventolin™

- participating in government run screening and treatment programs such as the biannual bowel screening program for the over 50s, having mammograms, Pap smears and regular prostate checks, and having childhood and seasonal influenza (flu) vaccinations.

For instance, 90 percent of all women who develop cervical cancer in Australia have either not had a regular Pap smear or have not had one at all.

Other medical illnesses such as diabetes require you to be a diligent and active participant in the monitoring and management of your own condition on a daily basis. It is incumbent on you to play your part in doing this.

The other way you can help your regular upfront fee paying GP is to help them financially. This you can do by attending their practice for all consultations, rather than attending a bulk billing

GP for short consultations. Short consultations can be the financial lifeline for some general practices. If GPs can claim for consultations that take less time than that allocated for them by Medicare, they will have more time for patients who take longer. The only time when this should not apply is when you are really sick and cannot afford to go to see your fee paying GP. Do not forgo seeing a doctor if you really need to just because you cannot afford to do so. In this circumstance see a bulk billing GP or go straight to the emergency department of your local hospital, if your condition allows. Alternatively, call an ambulance.

SO YOU NEED FURTHER TESTS OR INVESTIGATIONS

Planning for possible further tests or investigations

If your GP thinks your presenting medical condition warrants further investigation, she will organise for you to have some tests. These can vary from simple blood tests to x-rays and scans. Your GP will organise for these tests to occur by writing or printing out a pathology request or referral form which you will need to take with you.

These tests and investigations will help to determine:

- if there is anything wrong with you
- how bad your medical condition is
- if you need follow-up treatment with a specialist or even admission to hospital.

They can also act as a guide as to how long you can wait for this to occur.

Prepare for this consultation in advance by having something with which to write down the name of these tests and/or the specialist your GP wants you to see.

Consider going with someone who can do this for you if you are a little forgetful. This is because an increasing number of investigations are performed in different medical centres within the same building, and these centres often share the same receptionist. Consequently, the receptionist you call will not necessarily know which centre to direct your call. She will invariably ask you what investigation you are having or who you are coming to see.

Arranging tests or investigations

If your GP wants you to have tests or investigations, you must consider prioritising this appointment. Often it is important to have these tests and investigations done as soon as possible. Consequently, it is important to be flexible.

A number of these medical investigation centres offer the same service in a number of different geographical areas.

If you are prepared to travel out of area you can often attend on the day of your choice. Alternatively, you can opt to be on a cancellation list. This means you will make yourself available if the centre has a last minute cancellation.

Any unnecessary delay in having your investigations and potentially starting treatment may compromise your survival. IT IS AS SIMPLE AS THAT.

Following up on your results

If you ring the GP's practice for your results, ask the receptionist if they have received the results and if the doctor has seen them.

In most cases the GP indicates she has read the results by signing a copy of the report of the test results.

Some medical practices have a designated practice nurse whose role is to contact patients to let them know their results. Alternatively, arrangements will be made for you to attend the practice for your results.

Do not assume you will only be contacted if something is wrong with you. Check, even if this has been the usual practice in the past.

When you speak to your GP about your results, either in person or over the phone, make sure she has the results in front of her when she is speaking to you and is not simply relying on her memory of what she thinks the report said.

Case study

In 2003, Patient A was treated for breast cancer. In 2009 she developed pain in her left shoulder. She went to a medical centre where she saw Dr. B, who had been aware of her earlier diagnosis of breast cancer.

Dr. B referred Patient A for an x-ray and ultra sound scan of her shoulder. On completion of the x-ray and the scan, a specialist radiologist reviewed them. He noted that Patient A had a torn tendon which he attributed to the metastatic spread of the breast cancer into the woman's shoulder.

The radiologist contacted Dr. B and recommended Patient A be referred for a bone scan and be reviewed by an oncologist (cancer specialist).

A week later, Patient A went back to see Dr. B for her results. Dr. B informed her that she had torn tendon which he attributed to a sporting injury. He gave her a steroid injection. Patient A found this to be "excruciating". Dr. B failed to mention the radiologist's opinion that the pain was attributable to the spread of her breast cancer into her shoulder.

Patient A continued to experience pain in her left shoulder and went back to see Dr. B on no less than two other occasions.

Eventually, Dr. B referred Patient A to an orthopaedic specialist in 2010. The orthopaedic specialist diagnosed Patient A's breast cancer had spread to her shoulder. Patient A subsequently died in 2014.

This matter was referred to the Health and Disability Commission in New Zealand for investigation. In his defence, Dr. B told the inquiry he "either overlooked or completely forgot about the radiologist's comment in relation to a suspicious lesion". The radiologist's opinion would have been on the report of the test results that Dr. B had received.

Adding an extra check and balance

As an added safety measure, I have made an arrangement with my GP to receive copies of my blood results. She has facilitated this by writing for this to occur on the referral forms. Without my GP's written authorisation I would not be able to receive a copy of my results. I do this so I can check the results myself.

If you can read or understand English (or you have someone

who can do this on your behalf) and can compare numbers in the case of blood results, you can ask your GP to do this on your behalf. This is because all blood tests have a bracketed 'Reference' range of what is considered to be normal printed to the far right of each individual result.

Most pathology companies indicate when a particular result is abnormal by printing an asterisk (*) alongside the individual test result. Therefore you can see at a glance when something is abnormal. If you have had tests with this particular pathology company in the past, the most recent blood test results will usually be in **bold** print.

Date	10/04/07	**12/01/15**	Reference
Haemoglobulin	135	**128**	(119–160)

If a particular result has been ordered and is 'pending', make sure you follow up on this result with the pathology company or with your GP.

If there is an identified abnormality with your results, ask your GP for an explanation as to why she thinks you have an abnormal result and what it could mean for you.

If your GP considers the abnormality to be insignificant (not all abnormal results are significant), consider asking the GP to organise for the test to be repeated at a later date.

Even if your results are within the 'normal' reference range, check to see if your GP needs to discuss the results with you.

If your GP is assured of your need for further treatment for your medical condition, she will formulate a provisional or actual diagnosis for you and may refer you on to a specialist. She may even send you straight to the emergency department of your local hospital.

Getting a second opinion, and trusting your intuition

You can get a second opinion (or any number of opinions) at any time during the preliminary investigation phase with a GP or with a specialist, or during the treatment phase of your medical condition. A second opinion, as the phrase suggests, involves getting a second opinion as to your presenting medical condition from another doctor.

You should always consider seeking a second opinion if:

- you have any doubt about the reliability of the information provided by your doctor

- you lose confidence in any of your treating doctors

- you have signs and symptoms that remain unresolved or untreated

- your intuition tells you to do so.

Do not discount or ignore your intuition or deride the intuition of others.

Case study
Two-year-old Frankie Prebble had a small pink spot on her arm which began to grow and later started bleeding.

Her parents took her to three doctors before it was correctly diagnosed as a melanoma (a very dangerous skin cancer).

Her mother Michelle was quoted as saying: "If there's anything unusual that crops up on their child's skin, just get it checked out, and even if you've still got this feeling that it's not right, go get another opinion, and even another opinion." (Sydney Morning Herald (SMH): 12 October 2014.)

CHOOSING THE RIGHT SPECIALIST AND THE RIGHT HOSPITAL

Choosing the right specialist for your medical condition and the right hospital to which you are admitted are other crucial stages in the process of protecting yourself as a patient. It is crucial in terms of having a successful outcome to your treatment, reducing the risk of adverse events occurring, and potentially prolonging or saving your life.

Choosing the right specialist

If your GP is of the opinion you require specialist follow-up, she will make a recommendation as to the specialist she thinks you should see. This recommendation will invariably be based on the specialists she knows and with whom she has an ongoing professional relationship. They will generally be specialists in your local area.

If your GP recommends you see a specialist, ask her directly if your condition is life-threatening and how long you can delay before seeking a specialist's opinion. If your condition is not life-threatening, you have time to do some research into which specialist it would be best for you to see. Ask your GP, friends or relatives who they would recommend you see, and why.

If your GP refers you to someone with the same name as her

beware. She may be referring you to her spouse or cousin. This person may not be the best specialist for you given your particular medical condition, the urgency of your need for treatment, whether you want to be treated as a public or private patient, and their particular skill in dealing with your problem. Ask her why she is referring you to this particular specialist and what she knows of their experience in this area.

Be particularly careful if the plan is to admit you under the care of a specialist in a regional or rural centre, especially if they are known to be inexperienced in the particular speciality you require. This is because some of these specialists are professionally pressurised to perform procedures outside their field of expertise simply because there is no one else to do them. Others can have had limited experience of performing certain procedures.

You may be better off staying with friends or relatives and seeking treatment from specialists in a large regional town or in a metropolitan city instead. If in doubt, ask the specialist about their level of expertise and vote with your feet if they appear hesitant or if you are unsure.

If you are to be admitted to hospital for an elective procedure (not an emergency), and there is time to choose when you are admitted to hospital, find out from the specialist's receptionist if she will be there during the entire post-operative period before you make the appointment. For instance, you might want to avoid being admitted to hospital in the lead-up to Christmas in Australia. This is because many specialists go on annual leave during this period and will not be available for consultation should anything go wrong.

If the specialist you are referred to is particularly skilled in their field of expertise, they will usually have a long waiting list. If you want to see this specialist as a public patient, and if they do see patients as public patients (not all of them do), you may have to wait to see them.

If your medical condition is potentially life-threatening this could be too long. You can potentially see her sooner if you opt to see her as a private patient. You do not need private health insurance to see a specialist privately. You can pay the specialist directly.

I have to say at this stage this is not a plug for private health insurance. I do not have private health insurance myself, believing as I do that the public health system is as good, if not better than a lot of private hospitals in terms of the standards of medical and nursing care and speedy access to post-operative medical care. I am just being honest. How I deal with this is that I have an emergency fund set aside should I ever need to see a specialist quickly. In my opinion, it can be far cheaper than buying ongoing health insurance.

Another example of why a specialist may not be the best for you is taken from the speciality of orthopaedic surgery. It is no good obtaining a referral to see an orthopaedic surgeon for knee surgery if she spends nearly all her time doing hip surgery.

The specialist and her registrar will be up-to-date on the latest surgical techniques, artificial prostheses, and the specific allied health support required for hip surgery, but possibly not that for knees. If, for instance, you need knee surgery and your GP does not know an orthopaedic surgeon specialising in knee surgery, or there is not one in your area, strongly consider seeking treatment from one out of your area.

If your GP cannot recommend one, seek advice from family or

friends or do your own research if you can. Find out, for instance, who publishes research in the area of knee surgery. This can be found in the medical journals stored in medical research libraries, in major universities in your capital city. See who they cite in the reference pages of their journal articles as specialists in your area.

Just as it is with your GP, your professional relationship with your specialist is one you should honour.

Be wary if your specialist:

- does not listen to you

- makes rash and ill-informed judgements about you

- has not informed you of the side-effects of the medications she has prescribed for you

- has not informed you of the risks associated with the surgery she proposes to do for you

- has not physically examined you

- has done things without seeking your permission

- has done things which you think are inappropriate, or have made you feel uncomfortable.

If these things are of concern to you, and you cannot resolve them by talking them through with your specialist, talk this through with your GP and ask her to refer you to someone else.

This is especially important if the specialist has done things you feel are inappropriate or made you feel uncomfortable.

Case study

Patient A was referred to a gynaecologist for an opinion with regard to a lesion she had found on her labia.

As part of the examination process, she was asked to lie on her back on his consulting table with her legs apart while the gynaecologist sat between her legs and examined her.

While she was lying down, she heard the sound of a camera shutter button firing. She sat up to see the doctor holding a camera and making his way back behind his desk. She realised the doctor had taken a photograph of her genitalia without her consent.

While she knew he was probably taking a photograph as a 'before' and 'after' treatment record for his clinical records, she did not talk to the specialist in question about her concerns and she did not inform her GP. She simply vowed never to go back to see the same doctor if she needed any subsequent follow-up.

Case study

In April 2015, Dr David Wee Kin Tong, a former dermatologist, was sentenced to 18 months and deregistered as a doctor for the indecent assault of five female patients on the pretext of examining them for skin lesions at two skin cancer centres.

One woman presented with what she regarded as being suspicious looking moles on her right breast, collar bone and chin and Dr. Tong took photographs of her genitals.

With regard to a specialist's communication skill, you have to weigh up what is important to you. I, for one, would rather a brilliant technician when choosing a heart surgeon than one who is overly sensitive and a particularly good communicator.

While a referral letter is needed to see a specialist initially, additional referral letters are not required if your subsequent visits occurs within a year of the first visit. If you need to see the specialist after this time you will need a new referral letter from your GP. While this is true for Australia it may be different in other countries.

Should your specialist be of the opinion you require surgery, be wary if she asks you to sign a disclaimer before she agrees to operate on you. This disclaimer is designed to obviate the surgeon of any legal responsibility should anything go wrong with your surgery. If you sign this disclaimer you will have little recourse to legal action should anything go wrong during your operation.

Consider boycotting any specialist who undertakes this practice. Certainly check if this will be required of you from the specialist's receptionist before you obtain a referral to see the specialist from your GP.

If you forget to do this when you make an appointment to see the surgeon, and you are asked to sign a disclaimer before your operation, you can still choose not to do so. You can do this even if you are asked to sign the disclaimer at the theatre entrance.

However, this may mean your operation may be cancelled, even at this late stage, and you may not be able to have your surgery with this particular surgeon in the future.

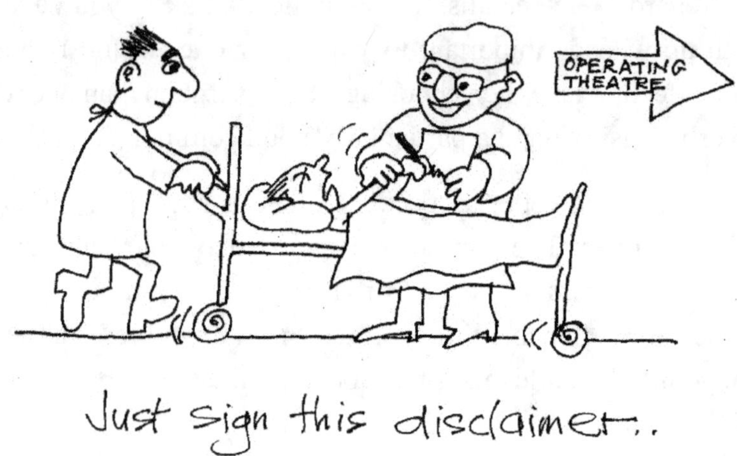

If you have occasion to see a specialist, seek to have them provide an update to your general practitioner after the consultation. This is especially important if you have any procedures performed.

I saw a colorectal surgeon in 2012, during which he performed a colonoscopy and took some biopsies. While he told me my colonoscopy was clear at the time, he was not able to tell me the result of the biopsies. I only found out in 2015 he had not informed my GP of the results of either the colonoscopy or the biopsies, and she had been unaware biopsies had been taken or that I had even had my colonoscopy.

Choosing the right public hospital

While the standard of medical and nursing care is generally good in all public hospitals in Australia, certain hospitals have a well-deserved reputation for their specialisation and expertise in certain medical fields. This is primarily because of their location and their access to differing amounts of public and privately generated funding for research with which they recruit and retain the top specialists in the field.

Unfortunately for some patients, this can have unforeseen, tragic and ultimately preventable consequences. An example of this is what occurs at a well-known inner city public hospital in Sydney at times.

This hospital has a well-known national reputation for its cardiac surgery. When I worked as the triage nurse in the emergency department of this hospital, it was not unusual for a person to pull up in the car park with a formerly living relative in the back of their car, having bypassed several excellent tertiary referral hospitals just to get to this hospital for treatment.

On another occasion, a middle-aged man drove all the way up to Sydney from Melbourne with chest pain. This is a journey of almost 1,000 kilometres and chest pain can be indicative of someone having a heart attack. Fortunately for him he was not having a heart attack. If he had been having one at the time, he most certainly would have greatly reduced his chances of surviving from it and probably would have died en route.

It is better to call an ambulance and have yourself taken to the nearest tertiary referral hospital than risk your life driving to your preferred hospital of choice. Plus, the treatment of a number of medical conditions including heart conditions has largely been standardised across all public hospitals in

Australia, as it has been in most first world countries. This means you can expect to receive the same treatment as everyone else for certain medical conditions, irrespective of which hospital you are treated in. This will be so, unless this proposed treatment requires you to give informed consent.

For those of you who are prepared to seek treatment from a public health specialist out of your area, there are other options. Here in New South Wales (NSW), in Australia, there is a person whose job it is to reduce the number of people on public health waiting lists. She is employed by NSW Health's Surgery Access Line and is called the Patient Access Co-ordinator. Her role is to advise you which public health specialists have the shortest waiting lists in NSW.

If you are prepared to be treated and followed-up in another part of the State you can often be treated earlier. This can be shorter still if you are prepared to accept a last minute cancellation.

Ring the health department in your State or Territory to see if they have such a person too. And remember, if someone is employed as a specialist in any public hospital in any metropolitan city, you can be assured they are excellent. These positions are much sought after and the selection process is very competitive and rigorous.

Should you be admitted to a public hospital and you have private hospital insurance, you might want to elect to be treated as a private patient.

If this is what you decide to do, you may want to negotiate with the public hospital that they pay for all of your 'out-of-pocket' costs in exchange for you being admitted as a private patient. Out-of-pocket costs are such things as the difference between the fee charged by the surgeon and the amount provided for that surgeon by your private health insurance company. Financially, this will be good for you and good for the public hospital.

Choosing the right private hospital

When it comes to private hospitals, this is a whole different ball game. Any doctor can set up shop in a private hospital with the agreement of the Board of that hospital. Selection in private hospitals is sometimes made on the basis of personal or professional relationships or the money they can bring to the hospital, rather than on merit.

You will not gain entry to the private hospital of your choice unless your specialist has what are called 'admitting rights' to that hospital. That is, the right to admit you to that hospital. So, if your heart is set on going to a certain private hospital for your medical treatment, you will need to check which specialists have admitting rights to the hospital and if your procedure can be done there.

If the specialist is more important to you than which private hospital you are admitted to, you will have to check which private hospital your preferred specialist has admitting rights to and go there. You should do this before you obtain a referral from your GP.

Not all procedures can be done in all private hospitals, some medical procedures cannot be done in any private hospitals, and some procedures are done, and arguably should not be done, in some private hospitals. This is because some private hospitals do not offer on-site and after-hours medical care, and most private hospitals do not offer intensive care facilities for their patients.

This means, if things start to go pear-shaped in private hospitals as they sometimes do, the best you can expect to happen is to be transferred to the nearest public tertiary hospital via an ambulance.

As you can imagine, this is not an ideal situation for any patient. You might want to reconsider having an anaesthetic in a private hospital if you have ever had an adverse reaction to an anaesthetic or you are having an anaesthetic for the first time. And you might also want to consider not having any surgery or procedure that is considered to be 'major' in a private hospital that does not offer on-site medical care 24 hours a day. This is because waiting for the ambulance to show up, load you onto an ambulance trolley, and transfer you to the nearest tertiary referral hospital could be the most perilous journey of your life.

Keeping yourself safe in a private clinic

An increasing number of surgical procedures are now being performed in private clinics, private rooms or in GP's surgeries. While the majority of these are quite safe, there are some safeguards you should insist on (see over for checklist for private clinics).

While it is important to insist on safeguards to ensure your safety while in private clinics, it is also important to adhere to the clinic's recommendations following your discharge home. For instance, if the clinic insists you be picked up after your procedure or have someone stay with you overnight when you are discharged home, ensure this occurs.

Under no circumstance should you say you have someone to drive you home or to stay with you overnight if this is not true, and the clinic is of the view it is important for you to do so. This is because some of the procedures are quite invasive and complications can and do arise at times. These may not be apparent on your discharge.

Similarly, after sedation or an anaesthetic, you are not able to drive or drink alcohol and you should not sign any legal documents.

Checklist for private clinics

- If you have ever had an adverse reaction to an anaesthetic or are having an anaesthetic for the first time, consider not having the procedure done in a clinic.

- Find out what drugs are going to be given and what effect they will have on you. If the drugs will make you semi-conscious or forgetful, ask the doctor to provide a chaperone. Alternatively, take a friend in with you and if appropriate to do so.

- Ask the doctor what she intends to do if she finds out you are having an adverse reaction to the drugs.

- Find out if you will need someone to collect you in a car, and/or to stay with you overnight after the procedure. If so, make sure these people will be available to do so.

- Ask the doctor what the potential risks could be for this procedure.

- Ask what she intends doing with the results if there are any, and follow up if necessary.

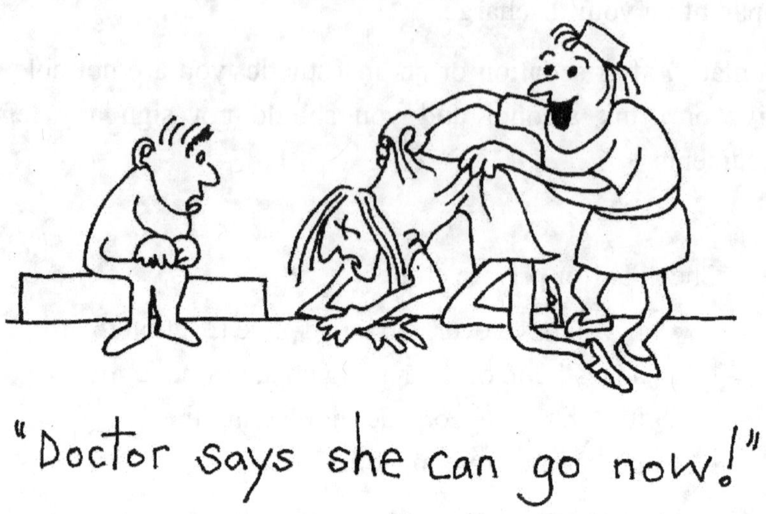

PREPARING FOR YOUR ADMISSION TO HOSPITAL

Unless you are admitted to hospital as an emergency patient, you will have plenty of time to prepare for your admission to hospital. The preparation you make before your admission to hospital will help to ensure the success of your admission.

The GP's referral letter

If your GP thinks you should see a specialist or should go to hospital, she will usually write a referral letter for you. This referral letter will usually contain a brief outline of your presenting medical problem, your medical history, a list of your current medications and the results of investigations and tests you have had to date, if any. If your GP has not prepared a referral letter, ask her to do so.

Take your personal medical file and your referral letter with you to the hospital.

The medications the GP has documented for you in the referral letter will usually be the scheduled medications that are prescribed for you while you are in hospital, unless of course it is thought that one of these medications is causing your illness. Often this will not be checked with you before they are prescribed, dispensed and administered to you in hospital. This is why it is extremely important to have a GP who is familiar with your entire medical history and the medications you are on, and for you to read the information supplied by her in the referral letter if possible.

The Admission Form

If you are to be admitted to hospital as an elective rather than as an emergency patient, you will normally be sent a pre-admission form to fill out. This form will again ask you to outline such things as your current medications and medical illnesses, known allergies, and past medical history. This form will be sent to you in advance of your admission so you will have time to think about the questions that need to be asked of you and to remember your medical history.

While it is important to fill in the form so you have your medical history clear in your own mind, do not assume any doctor and nurse will read it on your admission to hospital. Do not assume they will read it even if they take it from you.

If I could only have a dollar for every patient who has ever said: "But I wrote that on my admission form", when they subsequently find out a medication has not been prescribed for them, I would be completely retired by now.

Take it from me, doctors and nurses are notoriously poor at reading any handwritten information supplied by patients. They seem to solely rely on information supplied in the referral letter or given orally by the patient at the time of their admission. Despite this, when the hospital doctor admits you to the hospital and asks you for your medical history, refer them to your completed pre-admission form. Highlight any inconsistencies that may exist between what you have written on your pre-admission form and what appears in the referral letter.

If not specifically asked for it on your pre-admission form, add your weight and height to the form and ask the doctor who admits you to hospital to document these in your progress notes. If you require surgery or a procedure that requires an anaesthetic or sedation, have your weight added by the anaesthetist to the anaesthetic form and by the nurse to your pre-operative form.

To ensure the accuracy of the recording of your weight, take off all your clothes and weigh yourself after you have opened your bowels and passed urine in the morning, and before you have had your breakfast.

On no condition should you understate or overstate your weight.

Try to provide these measures in metric (centimetres and metres; grams and kilograms) rather than in imperial measures (feet and inches; pounds and stones).

If you weigh over 150kgs, most home and hospital scales will not accommodate your weight. You will have to organise to be weighed by a specialised weighing service. You may want to try a freight delivery company.

There was a time when all patients were weighed and had their height recorded on their admission to the hospital by the nursing staff, but this does not seem to occur to the same extent now. These measures are important for a number of reasons. They:

- govern how much anaesthetic and other medication you may need, if any

- provide an overall picture of your general health

- highlight problems you may encounter post-operatively and during your recovery in hospital

- act as a guide as to the type of allied health support you may need during your admission to hospital to obtain the optimal level of recovery in the shortest possible time.

What it means to give 'Informed Consent'

Before you have certain procedures and any operations in hospital or in private clinics you will be asked to sign a consent form. Your signature on the consent form is usually obtained by the specialist in her rooms if it is to be an elective admission, by a doctor in the emergency room if you are admitted to hospital as an emergency patient, or by a doctor on the ward if you are already an inpatient.

This poses a particular a problem for patients from CaLD backgrounds. While some doctors will take a risk and treat you even though they know you do not fully understand English and thus cannot give informed consent, others will not. Consequently, you may miss out on much needed treatment. This is why it is important in an English speaking health system for you to be able to speak and understand English, or at the very least have someone who can do so on your behalf.

The hospital can facilitate your understanding by engaging the services of the government health translating service. This is a free service, and can be used 24 hours a day, seven days a week.

If you do not know what operation or procedure you are having, or what the major side-effects of this operation or procedure could be, consider delaying the signing of this form until this is fully explained to you in a language you understand. Do this, unless of course it is in an emergency.

Consent forms

When you sign a consent form giving a doctor permission to operate on you, perform certain procedures on you, or give you certain medications, your signature indicates:

- the doctor has explained the operation or procedure to you and you fully understand what has been explained to you

- the doctor has made you aware of the major risks or adverse side-effects of the operation or procedure they are about to perform on you, or the medication they are about to give you

- you agree the doctor can do other things to you in the event of an emergency, or under unforeseen circumstances.

Preparing early for your admission to hospital

Unless your family member is admitted to hospital as an emergency patient, there is usually plenty of time to prepare for their admission to hospital. For family members who are elderly or frail, and especially for those suffering with dementia, this needs to begin long before they are admitted to hospital and even if they live in care homes or in supported accommodation.

In my professional experience, many elderly patients admitted to hospital are underweight and clearly malnourished, while a large number are also under-hydrated or are clinically dehydrated.

There can be many reasons for this. It may be related to the clinical reason they are to be admitted, it may be due to other yet to be diagnosed clinical reasons, or it may be because they have not been given enough food or fluids. Alternatively it may be because they simply cannot manage to obtain these for themselves.

For people over the age of 50, their body's thirst sensation diminishes naturally and keeps diminishing with age. This is why many elderly people do not feel thirsty at all, even though they hardly drink anything.

I have learnt from past experience that just because someone is living in a large, beautiful home or in a nursing home does not mean they have the where-with-all to feed themselves properly or to get themselves adequate fluids, or that these have been given to them by the people charged with looking after them.

According to the media department of Hammondcare, at least 50 percent of people in nursing homes are either under-hydrated or are clinically dehydrated. One report they made mention of reported that more than 90 percent of patients admitted to hospital from nursing homes were under-hydrated or clinically dehydrated.

Do not assume that just because your Aunt Molly says that she has been eating and drinking properly in the lead-up to her admission to hospital she has in fact been doing so. It is clear, in the immediate lead-up to their admission and perhaps for quite a while before hand, many elderly patients have not been eating and drinking properly.

If you know such a friend or relative is going to be admitted to hospital, consider at least visiting or staying with them for a while before their admission to ensure they are eating and drinking properly. Consider doing this even if they are having a relatively minor operation. This is because their operation may be postponed, or your friend or relative may not have been properly assessed before their operation.

It does not take much for a person who has not been eating and drinking properly in the lead-up to their operation for them to quickly be in trouble during the post-operative period.

The complications that under-hydrated or dehydrated people encounter can range from constipation to more serious problems such as acute renal failure or the development of a deep vein thrombosis.

Consider giving your friend or relative high calorie and high protein enriched foods and plenty of fluids before their admission if there are no clinical reason such as diabetes or heart or renal failure for doing so. If in doubt, seek advice from their GP. This is because some patients may be on low protein and restricted calorie diets, while others may be on restricted amounts of fluids.

Many patients arrive without simple things such as their toothbrush, toothpaste and their slippers, and others without any prior knowledge of their own medical history or even the medications they are on. Many patients do not have, or do not know, the names of their regular GP(s) and cannot tell hospital staff where they practice. While arriving without a toothbrush or toothpaste is not important to a patient's recovery or survival from an operation, knowing what medications you are on or what your medical history is could be.

A checklist of what to bring with you into hospital

- ☐ A complete copy of your medical file (see above) and any recent scans and x-rays
- ☐ Your medications, especially any alternative, homeopathic, trial, unusual or time sensitive medications
- ☐ Your GP's referral letter
- ☐ Medicare card and health benefit card and/or details of your private health fund if applicable
- ☐ Glasses, dentures, hearing aids (spare batteries), CPAP machine
- ☐ Walking aids including a walking stick, a walking frame, or a four-wheeled walker
- ☐ A small amount of cash
- ☐ Nightwear, dressing gown, shawl

Checklist cont.

- ☐ Well-fitting slippers (no backless slippers) and rubber thongs or flip-flops
- ☐ Antiseptic gel, wipes and tissues
- ☐ Washing items: shampoo, soap, shaving foam, razors, toothpaste, toothbrush and hairdryer etc
- ☐ Soft comfortable pillow, eye shield, and ear plugs
- ☐ Mobile phone and charger and plug-in ear phones for the radio or television
- ☐ Books, magazines, knitting
- ☐ Thickening powder, if the specialist thinks you will have trouble swallowing after head or neck surgery or you have had a stroke (it thickens fluids such as water, coffee and soup and can be bought from a chemist or pharmacy)
- ☐ Previously dispensed anti-clot support stockings if you have them and if they are still in good condition and fit you properly
- ☐ Large pad and pens if there is a probability you will not be able to speak after surgery
- ☐ Your favourite night-time beverage such as hot chocolate, Milo or Ovaltine powder.

The advantages of being prepared mean you:

- can be medicated when necessary and not when the pharmacy re-opens
- can be medicated with alternative medications the pharmacy will not supply
- can help to keep yourself safe from falling
- do not share these items with other people and are not reliant on pre-used hospital stores
- can protect yourself from contracting infections
- get plenty of rest and sleep
- will have stockings that fit you properly and will be effective
- will be able to thicken plain water, and will not have to rely on hospital supplies.

Case study

One hospital that I have worked in only supplies thickened cordial and fruit juices to their patients who have swallowing difficulties and cannot drink thin fluids. They do not supply thickened water.

I have tasted these products and they are awful. I would not want to try and swallow these products on a regular basis.

As yet I have been unsuccessful in changing hospital practice, despite complaining. This remains a work in progress.

Chapter 2:
A patient in hospital

SAFETY FEATURES OF A THOROUGH ADMISSION PROCESS

Alternative treatments to admission or staying in hospital

If you are being admitted to hospital for the sole administration of antibiotics to treat an infection, and the hospital has a 24-hour community outreach program that provides such a service, ask to be referred to this service during the admission process instead of being admitted to hospital. You can also ask to be referred to this service if you are only staying in hospital for the administration of antibiotics.

Public hospitals are increasingly offering such a service as an alternative to admitting patients to hospital and to facilitating a patient's early return to work. This will invariably be more convenient for you and will reduce your exposure to infections. This is especially true if you are elderly and/or vulnerable to contracting other infections. Unfortunately, some doctors who work in hospitals are unaware of this service so will not know to offer it.

The different coloured bands on your wrist

All patients should be given an identity band to wear in hospital. This should occur as soon as they are taken in to see a doctor in the emergency department or they arrive on the ward. This should occur irrespective of how long they are to remain in the hospital.

> Coloured bands
>
> - White band – information about your identity, such as full name, date of birth, address and medical record number
> - Red band – information about any allergies
> - Green band – indicates you may be at risk of falls.

The identity band is usually white in colour and is usually worn on the wrist. The identity band usually contains information such as your full name, date of birth, address and medical record number (MRN).

If you are admitted to hospital, this identity band will be updated to include details of your treating specialist and the date of your admission.

Before this band is placed on your arm and/or leg, read it and make sure the details on the band are correct. If you have trouble seeing the band, ask the nurse to read it out to you. Pay particular attention to the spelling of your name and your date of birth.

On no condition should you accept the administration of any medications or intravenous fluids if you are not wearing an identity band, unless of course it is an emergency, and on no condition should you be in any hospital for any length of time without wearing an identity band. THIS IS VERY IMPORTANT.

Some hospitals place this information in a red band if you have any allergies, while other hospitals require you to wear a second red band detailing information about any allergies you may have.

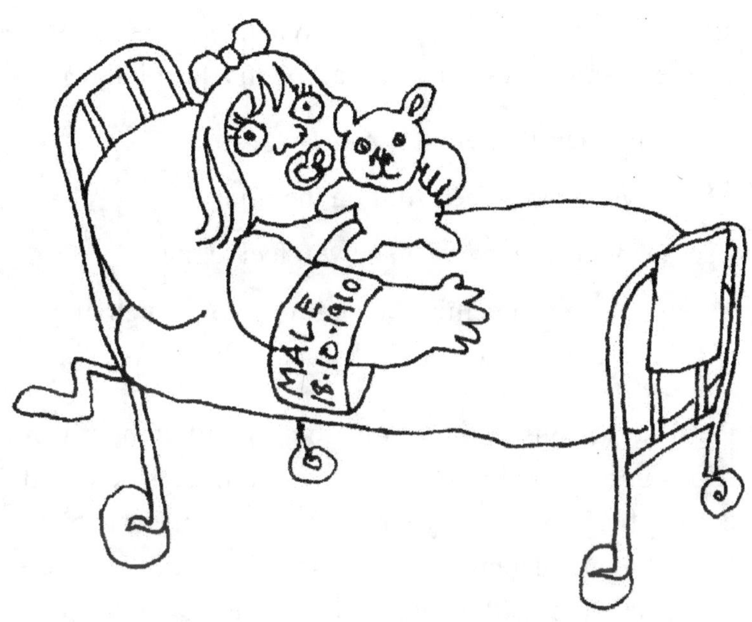

If you are assessed as being at increased risk of falls or your presentation or admission to hospital is precipitated by a fall, you may be required to wear yet another band. This is often green in colour. If in doubt, ask your primary nurse about the bands.

If for any reason any of these bands are cut off or fall off, contain information that is incorrect or incomplete, or you are transferred to another hospital, ask for this information to be updated and for new bands to be issued.

Falls prevention starts on admission to hospital

If you are elderly, physical disabled or visually impaired, and especially if you usually walk with a walking aid such as a stick or a four-wheel walker, do not make any attempt to get out of bed without a nurse's help until your ability to mobilise without assistance has been assessed. Do not attempt to get out of bed even if you see the nurse is too busy to help you when you need it. You are at an increased risk of falling in a hospital because:

- it is an unfamiliar environment for you

- things may have been spilt on the floor

- some medications can make you feel dizzy

- there may be something wrong with you which may make you uncharacteristically unsteady on your feet.

If one of the reasons you try to get out of bed without waiting for help is because you need to go to the toilet quickly, and the nurse is too busy to answer your call immediately as is often the case, ask for an incontinence pad to wear while you are in hospital. These are readily available for your use in hospital.

Finally, if you have ever:

- felt dizzy when you walk

- nearly fallen in the past

- fallen at home or out in the street

- needed to walk with a walking stick, walking frame or four-wheeled walker

and you have not been specifically asked this information by the nurse who admits you to hospital, volunteer this information. Volunteer this information, even if you have long accepted falling over as a 'normal' feature of everyday life.

Medical admission process

If you are admitted to hospital as an elective patient, you will be admitted straight to the ward. There, the junior doctor from the admitting team will take your medical history, examine you, order your blood tests, and arrange for any further investigations deemed necessary such as a chest x-ray or a scan.

When the doctor asks you for your medical history, refer them to your pre-admission form, your personal medical file and to the GP's referral letter if you have one. This will help to ensure the doctor has all the necessary information. As an added safeguard, show her any medications you have brought in with you from home.

Emergency department admission

If you require admission via the hospital's emergency department, there is a likelihood you will not have the things you need to keep you safe while you are in hospital. This is especially true if you are brought in by ambulance. Refer your friends or relatives to the 'What to bring with you into hospital checklist' and have these items brought in for you.

The nursing admission process

When you are admitted to hospital you will have your observations taken. This is usually performed by a nurse on the ward or the triage nurse in the emergency department. This usually involves taking your blood pressure, heart rate, temperature and blood saturation levels electronically via an 'observation (obs) machine' and visually counting your respiration rate.

If the nurse does not feel your pulse with her fingers or listen to your heart rate with a stethoscope, ask her to do so. This is because an obs machine will not necessarily pick up any irregularity in the rhythm of your heart rate, and this is an important piece of information for the doctor to know.

If you have had a mastectomy, ask the nurse to take your blood pressure on the arm on the opposite side of your body to where you have had the mastectomy. This means if you have had your right breast removed, ask the nurse to take your blood pressure on your left arm. This is especially true if you have had some lymph nodes removed. This rule should also apply to the insertion of an intravenous cannula.

Ask the nurse if your heart rate is regular. If it is irregular, then ask the nurse to organise for you to have an electrical trace of the rhythm of the heart (ECG) performed. This is a simple process which entails having sticky pads put on your chest and having these connected to a machine with wires. This is a pain free process, unless you have a hairy chest and the nurse has not thought to shave your chest first!

Participating in nursing assessments

If you are in hospital for any length of time and whether you are finally admitted to hospital or not, you will normally be asked to participate in a series of nursing assessments. These are designed to assess your risk of:

- falling in hospital
- developing pressure sores
- withdrawing from alcohol.

They will also be used to assess your general level of health and the possible need for allied health support while you are in hospital and following your discharge from hospital.

Be honest with your answers, especially when asked about your daily alcohol consumption. This is because you can become quite confused and disorientated when alcohol is suddenly withdrawn from you, such as occurs when you are admitted to hospital. As a result, you can be easily misdiagnosed as having something else wrong with you.

The hospital needs to know in advance if this is likely to occur so special monitoring can be started and certain medications can be prescribed for you. This will enable your nurse to quickly give you this medication should you suddenly start withdrawing from alcohol.

If you are not asked about your alcohol consumption, and you drink more than two standard drinks a day, inform the nurse who admits you to hospital.

The nursing care plan and its inherent limitations

During the nursing admission process on the wards, the nurse will formulate a nursing plan for you once you are admitted to hospital. The nursing care plan is an important legal document that governs how nurses will look after you or your relatives as patients in hospital. Unfortunately, it is one of the most poorly crafted and under-utilised documents in nursing practise.

For the most part the nursing care plan is a very basic document that is largely generic within the hospital. It is not standardised across hospitals and only covers the bare minimum of detail.

Even though it is a legal document, the nursing care plan is often not filled in properly and with enough detail for anyone to look after even the most basic needs of the patients. It does not serve to capture any of the idiosyncratic behaviour or care needs of patients at all.

The nursing care plan is particularly poor when used for patients with intellectual and physical disabilities or for those with complex care needs.

To these patients and/or their carers I would say only one thing: draft your own nursing care plan, update it when necessary, and give a copy of it to the nursing staff for use during your admission. If you do not do this you are going to spend a lot of time explaining to each and every nurse or doctor who looks after you or your relative how to do so properly. There is no reason why a nursing care plan you design cannot be used in conjunction with the hospital's nursing care plan to look after you as a patient.

Information to volunteer

If you are to be admitted to hospital and you have not had a bowel motion since the day before your admission, volunteer this information to the nurse who admits you to the emergency department or to the ward. What you want to avoid is becoming constipated while you are in hospital.

Periods of inactivity, dehydration, a lack of food and certain medications can make constipation much worse, and very quickly. The nurses need to know if this is a possibility as soon as possible.

If you normally take laxatives at home or certain foods to facilitate bowel motions such as prunes, and these have not been prescribed for you by your GP or supplied to you in hospital, inform the nursing staff so they can be, and if appropriate to do so.

Seeking a routine urinalysis

A urinalysis used to be routinely done for all patients when they were admitted to hospital. This test is simple and painless and is usually performed by the nursing staff. It involves collecting a urine sample into which the nurse dips a urinalysis stick.

A urinalysis stick informs the nurse if you have glucose, protein, blood, bile, ketones, nitrites or leucocytes in your urine, and provides information as to the pH or specific gravity of your urine. Such testing can provide an immediate indication as to your general health and can highlight other health problems which may be affecting you.

A urinalysis is something you should ask a nurse to perform for you while you are in hospital, even if it is not routinely offered to you. Do not be fobbed off if the nurse says you do not need a urinalysis. It is a simple thing for a nurse to do and can save you problems down the track. Ask the nurse to let you know the results after it has been performed.

If you are asked to provide a sample of urine for a urinalysis and you think you may have a urinary tract infection, inform the nursing staff so you can be given a sterile container into which you can pass urine. This will enable the nurse to send this off to pathology for testing if an infection is clinically indicated, and will ensure you are treated in a timely manner.

Requesting a routine blood sugar level

Pre-diabetes and diabetes is on the rise in Australia. Many people are unaware they have these conditions. If you find you:

- get dizzy

- become irritable if you do not eat regularly

- need to drink lots of water

- have a tendency to pass a lot of urine and have unexpectedly started wetting your underpants or your bed

ask for a routine blood sugar level to be performed.

Always ask for this test to be performed if you know you have these conditions, if you have been drowsy, or if you have had a period of unconscious. Do this even if you have been admitted to hospital with another medical condition. Again, it is a simple test. It is easily performed by nursing staff and involves pricking a finger with a lancet or small metal needle.

Pre-existing wounds or sores on your body

If you have any kind of sore or wound on your body arising from an injury or infection you have sustained or contracted before your admission to hospital, inform your nurse and/or attending doctor who admits you to hospital. Do this even if it is unrelated to your presenting medical condition.

Make sure someone looks at the wound and takes a wound swab if it is oozing fluid. If it is oozing fluid, make sure it is cleaned with normal saline (salt water). It may also need to be swabbed with an antiseptic solution and be covered with a sterile dressing.

You may be asked to consent to having the wound photographed on admission. Give your consent. This will serve as a record of the wound. If the wound is infected, you may need treatment for the infection during your admission or you may need to be isolated from other patients.

Once identified, the wound should be looked at on a daily basis to see how well it is healing. This should be done on a daily basis unless the nurse who is looking after you advises you otherwise.

If a community nurse has been attending to the wound before your admission to hospital, inform the nursing staff and ask for this service to be suspended while you are in hospital. Ask for the wound to be assessed by the hospital's wound clinical nurse specialist if such a person exists in the hospital in which you are admitted.

Preventing the spread of infections

Many patients who come into hospital have problems with their blood circulation in their legs or have difficulty with the feeling in their toes. Consequently, if they scratch their skin in response to the irritation of a fungus, they are at risk of developing a nasty infection in their skin. This may go unnoticed by the patient and their carers until it poses a serious and significant risk to their health.

If you have a fungal infection on the skin of your feet, inform the nursing staff so it can be treated while you are an inpatient. In addition, bring rubber thongs or flip-flops in with you and wear these at all times when using communal facilities.

If you know or suspect you might have any other kind of infection, or you have been isolated in a hospital in the past with an infection, inform the hospital in advance of your admission. Alternatively, inform the first nurse you see when you are admitted to the hospital. This will ensure precautions can be taken to protect you and other patients, and the hospital staff designated to look after you.

Schedule 4D and schedule 8 medications

If you normally take schedule 4D drugs such as Panadeine® Forte or Valium® or schedule 8 drugs such as oxycodone or OxyContin® at home, inform the doctor or nurse during the admission process.

If you have brought this type of medication into hospital with you, inform the nursing staff you have them. Be prepared to relinquish them for safe keeping in the ward's drug safe until your discharge, or until they can be given to a relative to take home for you. Alternatively, leave them at home in a safe place. This is because there are some unsavoury characters in hospitals, and they often seek to steal these types of drugs.

It is also important you do not take any of the medication you may have brought into hospital with you, without first informing the nursing staff.

Providing a medical history or translating on behalf of others

If you are going to elicit and provide a medical history on behalf of others it is absolutely imperative you provide the entire medical history asked of you and gathered from the patient, even if it is personally uncomfortable for you, or goes against your cultural norms to do so.

The doctor or nurse will not be asking questions to embarrass you or your relative. The questions asked of you and the patient are important and should be answered fully and truthfully.

If you are specially asked about your friend or relative's alcohol consumption or illicit drug use, say what you know to be true.

The doctor needs to know immediately if this is a possibility.

Many people drink a lot of alcohol and take illicit drugs in private, even when it may be illegal (under-age drinking is becoming increasingly common) or against their cultural beliefs to do so. Consequently, they can experience adverse side-effects such as confusion and hallucinations when alcohol or certain drugs are suddenly withdrawn from them in hospital.

It is not uncommon for people to present with delirium suggestive of a severe infection when they are simply withdrawing from alcohol. This is especially true of some elderly people.

It is not fair to, and can be dangerous for, a patient if you fail to ask them something the doctor needs to know. If the doctor has asked you to translate something and you do not want to do so, or you think it is not your place to do so, let the doctor know. As a general rule, do not act as an interpreter for any relative if there is time to seek an independent interpreter for them.

WHAT YOU NEED TO KNOW ON ADMISSION TO HOSPITAL

There are a number of strategies you can adopt when you are admitted to hospital to ensure your safety during your admission. Documented below are the main ones you need to know.

Playing your part in preventing or limiting the spread of infections

All people carry microbes on their skin, in their throat, or up their nose that can cause infections. While these microbes may not be harmful to you, they can be deadly to others. Therefore, the one thing I would ask is that you and your relatives play your part in limiting the spread of these microbes. This should be done in all public places, but especially in hospitals and in a GP's waiting room.

The things you can do include:

- If you are sick, do not visit a hospital as a visitor.

- If you are coughing or sneezing and need to go to see a GP or to visit a hospital, ask for a mask to wear. Do not continue coughing or sneezing in the waiting room or in a hospital without wearing a mask or at the very least covering your mouth with your hand or with a tissue. Sit apart from other patients.

- Use the antiseptic solution on display before you enter the ward, and wash and dry your hands properly before you enter your room, when you leave your room, after going to the toilet, after touching your undressed wounds or sores, before and after using any of the shared communal facilities such as the toilets, kitchen or the lounge, and before eating.

- Do not touch the food of other patients in the communal kitchen.

- Use tissues for blowing your nose or coughing up sputum and dispose of these in your waste bag or in the bin after each use. Do not use tissues more than once. If you do not have any tissues, ask the nurse for a box of tissues. If the box has already been opened, swab the top of the box with an antiseptic cloth before use.

- Do not share magazines, shampoos or conditioners with other patients without swabbing them first and afterwards with antiseptic solution.

- Do not sit on the beds or chairs of other patients.

- Do not use the blue gloves in boxes hanging above the sink.

- If you are using the communal commode chairs or walking frames, swab the hands of these devices with antiseptic lotion on a regular basis and wash your hands after use.

- Wear shoes or hospital issue non-slip socks on all occasions, and do not walk around the ward or to the toilet with bare feet.

- Consider bringing in rubber shoes such as thongs or flip-flops for use in the shower, and especially if you have a fungal infection on your feet.

- If you are required to stay on bed rest, ask for a bottle of antiseptic lotion with which you can clean your hands.

Quick guide to limiting the spread of infection

- If you are sick, do not visit a hospital as a visitor.

- If you are coughing or sneezing, wear a mask.

- Use the antiseptic solution on display.

- Do not touch the food of other patients.

- Use tissues for blowing your nose or coughing up sputum.

Setting and maintaining health care standards

In a Canadian study on a transplant ward in 2014, researchers found only:

- 30 percent of those people who had agreed to being tracked with wireless devices in a hand hygiene study washed their hands after a bathroom visit

- 40 percent washed their hands before a meal

- 3 percent washed their hands while using the communal kitchens on the ward or when they entered their own room

- 7 percent washed their hands when they left their room.

This has led researchers to conclude that patients themselves are at risk of infecting themselves and others.

While it is well known children are influenced by the standards demonstrated or set by adults, so are other adults. If someone sees you consistently:

- washing your hands before meals or after you have used the toilet

- using the disinfectant hand-wash before you enter or leave a ward

- using tissues when you sneeze or blow your nose or clear your throat

- wearing a face mask when you go to a GP's practice, visit a hospital, or travel in an aircraft

- wiping communal surfaces such as handrails in trains or entertainment consoles and tables in planes with antiseptic wipes they will be more likely to follow your example (or at least consider doing the same) in the future. This will have the effect of reducing your exposure to viral and bacterial loads and will help to create a safer environment for everyone, including both you and your family.

Maintaining health care standards

Just as you have a role in setting standards, you also have a role in maintaining and insisting on standards. As you become aware of what these standards are, you will be in a position to play your part in maintaining them. While I know it is difficult for patients to challenge health professionals, especially when it comes at a time when they feel less able to do so, it is important you do. Often you are the only one who sees a health professional breach the standards and it is important you speak up. It is alright to challenge doctors and nurses on their actions or lack of action.

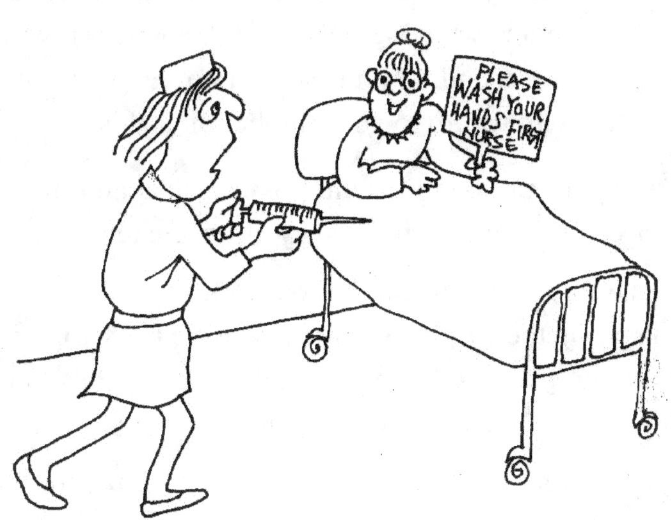

Not only will you be protecting yourself, you will be protecting others. If a health professional continues to breach the standards after you have pointed this out to them, ask to speak to the ward or unit's manager and raise it with them. Involve the infection control manager if the breach involves the potential spread of infection.

Your call button

My experience of the hospital call button system is this. The length of time a nurse will take to answer the bell will be proportionate to:

- the number of times you have rung it

- how sick the nurse thinks you were the last time you rang it

- what else is happening on the ward at the time

- how you respond to the nurse who responds to it.

If you keep ringing your bell for minor or trivial things, or you are rude to the nurse who does answer it, the longer it will take for the nurse to respond to your call button the next time. My advice to you with regard to your call button is this:

- Keep your call button within easy reach at all times, especially if you are in anyway incapacitated.

- Make sure that your call button works by either triggering the pager your primary nurse is wearing or the warning system on the ward, and ensure your call button works at the start of each new shift.

- Think through all the things you may need before you use the call button.

- Use your call bell sparingly and only when you really need to.

- Under no circumstance rely on the call button to summon help in a perceived emergency for yourself or for others. Instead yell "HELP, nurse" in a very loud voice. Keep yelling "Help, Help" until someone responds. This is also true of the emergency call button in the toilet.

Preventing a deep vein thrombosis (DVT)

One of the biggest causes of injury to patients is the development of blood clots in your vein. It is estimated that more than 14,000 people develop blood clots in a vein each year in Australia, and 5,000 of these die as a result. This is more than those who die of breast cancer, bowel cancer or from road traffic accidents.

The majority of people who develop blood clots are inpatients or recently discharged patients.

If you are in the emergency department for any length of time, and especially if you:

- are elderly

- are immobile in any way

- are likely to be staying overnight or will be admitted to hospital

- have not drunk anything for a while, are on restricted fluids, or are 'nil by mouth'

- have circulation problems in your legs

ensure you are wearing a pair of the hospital's thick white

support stockings (they may be a different colour in different countries).

Make sure these stockings are tight fitting and feel like they are putting pressure over the entire length of your leg. If these stockings are easy to pull on and up your leg, or do not come up to your knee in the case of 'knee-high' or to your groin if they are full-length stockings, they are not the right size for you. They will be ineffective and should be changed. Ask the nurse to measure your legs properly and change the stockings for the right size.

If the stockings become ruffled ask the nurse to pull them up for you. Most people who need support stockings should have difficulty putting them on and pulling them up themselves. It is OK to ask the nurse to do this for you. This is what would be expected of you.

While these stockings are uncomfortable to wear, do not forgo wearing them for any length of time for the entire time you are in hospital unless you have discussed this in advance with your doctor. Take these stockings with you on your discharge home. They cannot be reused for other patients. You can use them for subsequent admissions to hospitals, during long-haul flights, or in professions that require you to stand or sit for long periods of time. You can also use them if you are confined to bed for any period of time or sit for long periods of time.

If you arrive back from theatre and you are wearing calf compressors, ask for your nurse to attach these to a calf compressor machine. Calf compressors are designed to intermittently blow up with air, and to put pressure on the outside of your legs so as to usher the blood along inside the vein. These are not uncomfortable to wear.

Ensuring the right drugs are prescribed for you

The medications prescribed for you in hospital will normally be a combination of medications. This combination will depend on the reason why you are admitted to hospital and what has happened to you while you have been in hospital. The doctor may prescribe you medications:

- to prevent you from getting ill such as antibiotics

- to treat your new illness

- to stop the new illness from getting worse

- to offset the effects of other medications that have been prescribed for you (an example of this is laxatives, which are often prescribed to offset the effects of those medications that can slow down the bowel and make you constipated such as strong analgesia).

If you normally take medications at home, check to make sure these have been prescribed for you in hospital. In addition, make sure they have been prescribed for you in the right dose and at the right time of day.

If your medication is not given to you, has been given to you in a different form or different dose, or has been given to you at the wrong time of the day ask your primary nurse or doctor for an explanation.

Do not assume just because a medication has not been prescribed for you or given to you that your doctor does not want you to have it. Assume instead that a mistake may have occurred.

As a general rule, the doctor will usually prescribe your normal medication for your use in hospital unless of course she thinks this is the cause of your illness.

Taking your medication at the right time

If you know you should have certain medications like thyroxine an hour before you eat your breakfast, or diabetic tablets a half an hour before you eat your breakfast and your evening meal, do not start eating these meals before you have taken them.

The rules you have for taking these tablets at home will usually apply in hospital. Do not assume hospital staff know best, or they have reasons for doing what they do. Again, assume a mistake may have occurred instead. If you are in any way concerned about any of the medications prescribed for you in hospital, CHECK, CHECK and CHECK again.

Case study

Patient A was admitted to hospital. Following a nursing review of her clinical file eight days later it was discovered she had not been prescribed her usual daily dose of thyroxine. This is despite the fact her GP had documented this in her referral letter to the hospital.

There was also no mention that this omission had been mentioned by Patient A in the preceding eight days before the mistake was realised, even though the patient had been on the drug for the last 28 years and had only come into hospital with a broken leg following a fall.

It was not known why the patient failed to mention this omission.

Case study

Patient B was admitted to hospital. She had a past medical history of having had a heart and lung transplant for which she had been prescribed an anti-rejection drug. She knew she was required to take this drug on a daily basis to prevent her body from rejecting the transplanted organs.

During her admission for an unrelated condition, she was informed by a nurse one Friday that she was not going to be given her anti-rejection drugs until after a blood level had been taken for the drug on the following Monday.

Knowing the importance of taking this medication on a daily basis, Patient B queried this with the nurse and was assured this was correct.

Not satisfied with the nurse's explanation, and not having an opportunity to talk this over with her transplant team because it was the weekend, Patient B continued to take her own supply of the medication.

Patient B's concerns were realised when her team confirmed the nurse had misunderstood what was intended by the treating team. The patient had been correct to continue her medication.

Protecting yourself during the administration of medications

Medication errors are the most common form of injury suffered by patients in hospitals. Hospitals seek to protect patients from these errors by implementing a number of centralised and hospital-based policies and protocols. By informing you as to what should happen with regard to the administration of medications, I hope to help you to protect yourself as a patient from this type of error.

When health professionals are giving medications to patients they should follow certain protocols and procedures. These vary according to the type of medication that is given.

The most important of these protocols is the 'Five Rights'.

The Five Rights protocol

1   Right patient

2   Right medication

3   Right dose

4   Right route

5   Right time

You can help to reduce the possibility that mistakes with medications can occur by doing several important things:

- Be aware of how many medications you normally take and when, and what they look like. If you are about to be given too many tablets, unrecognisable medications, or at an odd time of the day, bring this to the attention of the administering person and ask for an explanation.

- Before accepting medications, make sure the administering person has verified your name, date of birth, and if you have any allergies. Make sure these are then checked against your identity band, your allergy band (if you have one), and your medication chart.

- Do not accept the administration of any intravenous, subcutaneous, intra-muscular or intra-thecal (in the spine) injections, or schedule 8 or schedule 4D medications such as morphine, OxyContin®, oxycodone, Panadeine® Forte, Valium®, or temazepam unless there are two people checking this information with you.

- Do not accept any medications left for you on your bedside while you were sleeping or away from your bed.

- Do take oral medications from a transparent syringe. These should be given in a red syringe in Australia.

Protecting yourself during the administration of intravenous fluids and drugs

During your presentation to the emergency department and/or admission to hospital, you will invariably need to have bloods taken, and you may need to be given intravenous fluids or medications. These fluids or medications will be administered directly into your blood stream via a cannula. A doctor or nurse will insert the cannula and take the bloods, while the nurse will usually administer the intravenous medications and fluids.

Damage to veins, infections arising from the insertion of intravenous cannulas, and complications arising from the administration of intravenous fluids and medications are common in hospitals and account for increasing rates of harm to patients.

These harms are for the most part preventable, and are usually the result of poor medical or nursing practice. By advising you of what should happen in hospitals when you are having a cannula inserted and/or when you are being given intravenous medications and fluids, I hope to help you to protect yourself against poor practices.

Inserting the cannula or a central line

Your intact skin is your greatest defence against contracting infection. If there are no breaks in your skin you will be at a low risk of contracting many hospital borne infections.

The insertion of a needle in your skin, and then the threading of a plastic cannula through your skin and into your vein, represents a major breech of your skin's natural defence. This puts you at increased risk of contracting an infection. This is especially true if it is preceded or proceeded by poor medical or nursing practices. It is also true if you have a pre-existing medical condition that puts you at increased risk of developing an infection. Therefore, before you allow anyone to attempt to put a needle into your skin you should ensure they have washed their hands before they start and cleaned your skin thoroughly with an antiseptic wipe or with antiseptic lotion. This is one of those times to be assertive, and it is all right to ask the health professional if they have done so.

While most health professionals will wear gloves when inserting peripheral cannulas, others may not. This is because it can be difficult to feel for a vein into which to insert a needle while wearing gloves. This is especially true for elderly patients whose veins lose their elasticity, or for those patients who have lost a lot of blood.

It may not matter if the health practitioner does not wear gloves when inserting a peripheral cannula as long as they have washed their hands properly before they start. However, a doctor should always wear sterile gloves when inserting a peripherally inserted central catheter (PICC) or a central line.

Ensuring the right location of the cannula

Before you allow the health professional to insert a peripheral cannula, ask them why they are putting it in. If it is just for taking blood, to give you one bag of fluid, or one dose of antibiotics, it probably will not matter where it is inserted.

If there is a likelihood you are going to need more than one bag of intravenous fluid, or the plan is to give you a number of doses of antibiotics that require admission to hospital, consideration needs to be given to the location of the cannula.

If you allow the health professional to insert the cannula in the crook of your arm (opposite side to your elbow) you are going to spend your entire time trying to keep your arm straight. You will need to keep your arm straight to avoid bending the plastic cannula in the vein in your arm and so obstructing the flow of the intravenous fluid.

If your intravenous line is attached to an electronic pump, this pump is going to alarm each time you bend your arm obstructing the flow of intravenous fluid, and it will drive you and others to distraction.

Importantly, it is also going to result in nurses coming to your bedside to fiddle or flush the cannula with normal saline. This will correspondingly increase the risk of you contracting an infection through the cannula or giving set.

You might ask why health professionals cannulate the veins in the crook of the arm when they can be so problematic. The answer is this: they are the easiest veins to access, and the person who inserts the cannula will not be the one trying to keeping the intravenous fluid flowing and has probably never had one themselves. So be warned.

If your condition is stable, and you are not receiving any intravenous medication or fluids through your peripheral cannula, ask your doctor if it can be removed. The longer a cannula is inside a vein, the greater the chance the vein will become infected.

The rubber bung or hub

Having inserted the cannula, the health professional will then screw a rubber sealed bung or hub into the cannula to prevent blood from leaking out of the cannula.

The hub will act as the port into which the intravenous line is inserted or through which intravenous medications are administered.

It is important the health professional anchors the hub with plastic, non-painful Steri-Strips and then covers the insertion point of the cannula through the skin with a transparent dressing.

Steri-Strips reduce the risk the cannula will be dislodged, and reduce the risk the insertion point will enlarge due to the friction of a hub that is constantly accessed and is not anchored properly. The transparent dressing ensures the insertion point of the plastic cannula remains visible.

Anchoring the cannula should always occur on the wards following admission, but is less likely to occur in emergency departments. This is especially true if the cannula is inserted in an emergency, the patient is only cannulated to obtain blood, and when treatment is likely to be limited. Despite this, I would encourage you to ask the health professional to anchor the line properly, irrespective of how much treatment you are to receive.

Anchoring the cannula properly

If you think you are likely to be staying in hospital or you are admitted to hospital, insist the health professional anchors the hub properly at the time of insertion and covers the cannula with a transparent dressing. In some hospitals, the health professional will then label the cannula with the sticker indicating the date the cannula was inserted and when it should be removed. This should be 72 hours after insertion. This cannula should then be looked at daily.

Make sure this cannula is removed after 72 hours and, if necessary, a new cannula inserted.

While the reinsertion of a cannula can be unpleasant for you, it will reduce the possibility of you contracting an infection through the hub or intravenous lines.

Exceptions are usually made for those patients who have poor or damaged veins and are difficult to cannulate, however, this decision will be made by the doctor.

If cannulas are left in for longer than 72 hours, it is even more important they are looked at every day.

Report any skin around the insertion point of the cannula that looks red or inflamed, is swollen or oozes, or is painful when knocked or accessed.

Administering intravenous medications

The nurse will choose one of four ways to administer intravenous medications to you:

- either directly through the hub connected to a cannula
- through the hub located along the intravenous giving set
- through the hub at the top of the burette attached to the giving set
- directly in the intravenous bag itself.

Principles for administering **intravenous** medications and fluids:

- No medications or fluid should be given intravenously in any vein that is red and inflamed, swollen, hot to touch or painful.

- The hub should be swabbed with antiseptic swab before inserting drugs or fluids.

- As a general rule, no medication should be given in an intravenous line containing Hartmann's solution without first flushing the line with normal saline and then flushing the line again after administration.

- No antibiotic should be given intravenously through a vein in less than two to three minutes because of the irritation it can cause veins.

- No antibiotic over 1gram should be given intravenously in less than 50 mls of intravenous fluid and administered in under 15 minutes.

- No intravenous antibiotic should be given to a patient for the first time, without the patient being given a small part of the dose to see if they are allergic to it first, before proceeding to give the rest of the dose.

- No intravenous medication should be given without two people performing the 5 Rights.

The mode of administrating the medication will be governed by the medication itself, the time over which it should be administered, or the protocol of the individual hospital concerned. For instance, some hospitals allow certain intravenous antibiotics to be given as 'a push' (as an injection directly through the hub in the cannula) over a period of two to three minutes, while other hospitals require these same antibiotics to be administered in 50 to 100 mls of normal saline and to be given over 15 to 30 minutes.

Whatever variation occurs in the particular hospital in which you are being treated, the principles remain the same for the administration of intravenous medications or fluids.

The danger in receiving intravenous fluids

If the plan is to give you intravenous fluids in hospital, this should be discussed with you in advance and ideally before they are administered. However, this usually isn't the case if you go to theatre for an operation. Most people are given at least one litre of intravenous fluids while they are in theatre, irrespective of the type of operation they have. Others are given much more.

Intravenous fluids are often continued in the post-operative period until patients are eating and drinking. This is why it is extremely important that you discuss with the anaesthetist who is going to administer this fluid to you during your operation, and may possibly chart more intravenous fluid for you after your operation, if you:

- have had any problems with your urinary tract system (kidney, bladder or ureters)
- have had any problem passing urine
- have dark urine

- have urine that smells

- have an enlarged prostate

- have swollen ankles

- are on 'water tablets' or diuretics

- have any trouble breathing

- need more than one pillow to sleep at night

- have had any problems with your heart in the past

- have had any abdominal operation

- have had any gynaecological procedure.

This should occur before your operation.

You will probably find the anaesthetist asks you questions related to these conditions before your operation, but may not do so if you are only having a minor operation. If in doubt, volunteer the information yourself and do so before your operation.

After your operation your primary nurse should check you have passed urine. If you cannot pass urine after your operation mention this to your primary nurse.

If you remain on intravenous fluids for whatever reason, monitor how much urine you are passing. If you seem to be receiving more intravenous fluid than you are passing urine, or you start experiencing difficulties passing urine, mention this to your primary nurse and have her measure your urine each time you pass urine.

It may be that you are simply dehydrated and need the extra fluid, or it could mean you do not have sufficient kidney function to excrete the excessive fluid as urine and you are becoming overloaded with fluid. This is a dangerous situation for you and you should act immediately.

Inform your primary nurse if:

- you do not seem to be passing enough urine
- you have difficulty passing urine, or you stop passing urine
- you develop chest pain
- you have any trouble breathing
- your sputum becomes frothy or
- your ankles become swollen or your feet become heavy.

If you cannot pass urine, or you do not seem to passing enough urine, ask your primary nurse to perform a bladder scan on you. The bladder scan should be performed immediately after you have tried passing, or have passed what little urine you can pass.

Even if you are not having intravenous fluids, you should be passing more that 200mls (glass full) of urine in an eight-hour period.

Pain

One of the ways health professionals assess the severity of your presenting condition, or any deterioration in your condition when pain is a factor, is to ask you to scale your pain from one to 10. Ten is the equivalent of being dropped off the tallest building onto concrete while 1 is a mere niggle.

You would be surprised by the number of people who scale their pain as being 10/10 when looking at you calmly, while half listening to the television or trying to conduct a mobile phone conversation. Do not exaggerate or downplay the amount of pain you are experiencing. This is because it may mean you are prescribed inappropriate medication, further unnecessary investigations or treatment may be ordered for you, or you may receive inadequate treatment.

Nurses should be asking you about your pain every day and, if you are in pain. They may ask you to scale the severity of your pain. If this is not happening, and especially if your pain is getting worse, suddenly gets worse, or you develop pain in a new area of your body, inform your primary nurse immediately.

If pain is:

- limiting your movement in bed
- hindering your ability to breathe in deeply or to cough
- limiting your ability to participate in physiotherapy and mobilise generally
- making the changing of dressings very unpleasant or
- seems inadequate for your needs

ask for your analgesia requirements to be reassessed and to receive analgesia in advance of any of these identified procedures.

Case study

Cultural aspects of assessing a patient's self-report of pain

Patient A presented to an emergency department of a large metropolitan hospital with a history of severe abdominal pain. She was on holiday from Northern Europe. Patient A was triaged and taken to a cubicle to wait for the doctor.

A Middle-Eastern doctor arrived to examine the patient. He asked her to scale her pain. The patient

scaled her pain as being 9/10. Patient A was sat up in bed at the time and did not appear to the doctor to be in much pain. Doctor B examined Patient A and decided to send her home without doing any further investigations.

During the night, Patient A's pain worsened.

Because she had already attended the emergency department and had been sent home, she decided to stoically stick it out over-night and to go back in the morning if she was still in pain.

According to her husband, Patient A started to vomit.

By the morning Patient A had collapsed and her husband called an ambulance. By the time Patient A arrived at hospital she was in septic shock from a perforated bowel and later died in hospital.

In his defence, the doctor justified his decision not to perform any further investigations and to send the patient home by explaining that, in his clinical experience of primarily treating Middle-Eastern patients, a patient who scaled their pain as being 9/10 would not normally be calmly sat up in bed.

In his experience, they would be flailing about in the bed or more likely walking about 'wailing' and demanding treatment.

He advised that he had not had any experience of treating northern European patients before and had not known their cultural reputation for personal stoicism.

If he had treated a northern European patient before, and one of these patients had scaled their pain as being 9/10, he would have known to book a theatre on route and almost certainly would have done more investigations before thinking about discharging them home.

Ensuring your safety equipment is checked every day

Behind nearly every bed in hospital is a patient's safety equipment. This normally includes two valves for the administration of oxygen and air, and a valve for suction. There is often a box at the back of the bed which contains two or more kinds of oxygen masks, oxygen tubing, suction catheters and a device called a Guedel airway.

Make sure this equipment is functioning on your admission and that this box is checked on a daily basis by nursing staff. If you see anyone taking any of the equipment from these boxes during your admission, seek to have it replaced as soon as possible. Ask this of your primary nurse and at a time when she is not too busy, or when there is an overlap of staff such as in the afternoon.

Pressure area sores

No one should develop a pressure sore in hospital or in a nursing home. A pressure sore is, as the name suggests, a wound or sore that develops on or in the surface of the skin as a result of prolonged and unrelieved pressure or friction on the skin. This pressure or friction causes the cells in the skin to die. Following the death of the tissue, the tissue breaks down and a sore or wound is formed.

While everyone is at risk of developing a pressure sore, some are at greater risk than others.

> People most at risk of developing pressure sores are those who:
>
> - are underweight
> - are largely immobile, such as people in traction, those who have had a stroke and those that have to sit up for long periods of time
> - are incontinent
> - have diminished feeling in their skin because of such things as peripheral neuropathy or a stroke
> - have fragile skin
> - are dragged up the bed with their skin rubbing across the sheets
> - are dying, and whose circulation is closing down
> - are lying on equipment or on a hard bed, such as those found in the emergency department.

While these sores can develop anywhere, they are more likely to form over bony prominences such as one's sacrum, heels and shoulders. This is why nurses will turn patients at regular intervals and reposition them. They will also organise for those patients considered to be at risk of developing pressure sores to be nursed on special pressure relieving inflatable mattresses, if appropriate to do so. This is all designed to reduce the pressure on the skin, and to reduce the risk of the patient developing a pressure area wound. They will turn patients from side to side even if they are dying.

Let the nurses turn you or the patient on a regular basis, even if it may be uncomfortable or painful for you to do so. If the nurses are not turning you on a two-to-four-hourly basis, even if you are on a pressure relieving inflatable mattress, ask to be turned. If you experience discomfort or pain when nurses turn you, organise to have some analgesia in advance of any planned turn.

If your skin feels like it is burning or is sore, and especially if this skin covers a part of your body which is constantly resting on the bed, ask the nurse to look at it. This may be the first indication that pressure needs to be relieved from your skin.

Pressure sores are often slow to heal, can be painful, and put patients at risk of contracting infections. They can greatly increase the amount of time a patient spends in hospital and so increases the risk of other complications occurring.

Be advised that the development of a pressure sore is considered to be indicative of poor nursing care and should not happen under any circumstances, unless of course a patient refuses to have their positioned changed or to be turned.

Knowing who your primary nurse is

At the start of each shift on general wards, a nurse is assigned to care for a group of patients. She will then become the 'primary' nurse for that group of patients. This means she will be responsible for organising and/or providing nearly all of the nursing care for that group of patients over the entire shift.

While your primary nurse is responsible for you while she is on the ward, she is not responsible for you while she is on her break. The responsibility for you at these times is assumed by one of her colleagues.

While some wards make a point of trying to ensure the continuity of care for their patients by assigning the same group of patients to the same nurses over the course of several shifts, others do not. This tends not to happen when the acuity (how sick a patient is and how much care they need) of the group of patients changes, the nurse has days off, or there is a challenging or difficult patient in the mix.

As there are three shifts in a day, you will have a three different primary nurses looking after you over a 24-hour period. There will be one in the morning, one in the afternoon/evening and one at night.

The morning nurse is responsible for you from about 7.30am and will continue to be responsible for you until their shift ends at approximately 3.30pm. This is when the afternoon/evening shift takes over and assumes responsibility for you until their shift ends at about 10pm. From approximately 10pm onwards, the nurse on night-duty is responsible for you. This will continue throughout the night until 7.30am in the morning when the morning shift takes over.

Making an ally of your primary nurse

It is important you establish who your primary nurse is for each shift. Ideally you should learn her name. Then, only address your concerns or queries to this nurse and not to any other nurses who may have occasion to care for you during the shift. This is true unless of course if it is an emergency. This is because it is this nurse who will:

- provide your care

- write in your progress notes

- communicate with your doctors

- make referrals for you

- give you your medications and monitor the effect these medications have on you

- arrange for your follow-up or additional care

- hand over details of your care and any problems you may be experiencing to your next primary nurse

- organise your discharge if she is looking after you at the time.

The fewer people directly involved with your care, the less opportunity there is for a mistake to occur or for things to be overlooked or forgotten.

The only times when this should not apply is when your primary nurse does not appear to respond to your concerns in a meaningful or knowledgeable way, when she has not taken action on your concerns, or when your primary nurse is a junior nurse.

Due to her relative inexperience, a junior nurse may not recognise the importance of your concerns or the problems that are troubling you. She may not act on them properly. In these circumstances it is important you ask to speak to the nurse-in-charge of the ward or to a doctor from your team. At the very least you should mention your concerns to the next experienced primary nurse assigned to look after you, if it can wait that long.

If your concern relates to your clinical presentation or treatment, then you should also inform one of the medical officers from your treatment team. This is because while the nurse may inform a member of your medical team and even write it down in your clinical progress notes, this does not mean it will be remembered by the medical officer, or that the nurse's clinical file entry will be read by the treating team. Some medical officers simply do not read nurses' clinical file entries.

On wards in metropolitan cities in Australia, you will share your primary nurse with four to five patients if it is during the day, and six to nine if it is at night. This is different in the acute or sub-acute sections of intensive care (ICU) where patients will have their own primary nurse if they are in the acute section, or share that nurse with one other patient if they are in the sub-acute section of ICU.

It is also different in hospitals in regional and remote areas where staffing is problematic. As you can imagine, this can vary from ward to ward and from hospital to hospital.

Staffing of wards depends on the acuity of the patients involved, the day-to-day employment availability of nursing staff, or the particular funding arrangements or practices of each hospital. Some hospitals staff wards according to the acuity level of the patients, while other hospitals staff wards according to the number of patients on the wards or the availability of nursing staff.

Staffing wards according to the number of patients is problematic. This is because you could be sharing your nurse's time with a number of very sick patients, the sickest of whom will assume most of your primary nurse's time. This will leave the bare minimum for you if you are not one of her sickest patients.

This is why you should support nurse union's attempts to introduce nurse-to-patient ratios in all hospitals. You do not want to be looked after by a nurse who has to look after a number of patients. This is when things can be over-looked or forgotten, or short-cuts taken. And you do not want this to occur at your expense.

Preparing for hospital-based investigations and procedures

The majority of investigations you have in hospital will require you to adhere to some kind dietary and/or fluid restriction before the procedure. These can vary from having nothing to eat or drink for up to four hours before the procedure, to not drinking coffee or eating chocolate, or only drinking clear fluids. Please adhere to these restrictions. If you fail to do so, for whatever reason, inform the nursing staff before you are taken down to the theatre for the procedure.

Final checking procedure before an operation

When you are taken to theatre for your operation, you are usually asked to undergo one last checking procedure before your operation. This usually involves the theatre nurse checking to make sure you are the right person, you have signed the consent form, and you know what operation you are having and where (for example, which limb).

If you are not asked this information for whatever reason, and you are in a position to do so, ask the theatre nurse who they are expecting to operate on and ask them what operation they intend performing.

If you have eaten or drunk any fluid after the time you were asked to refrain from doing so, this is the last time to 'fess up' and say so. It is critical you do so. It is better that your operation is delayed for a few hours than it is for you to have an anaesthetic at this time. You run the risk of aspirating or breathing in contents from your stomach down in your lungs. If this happens it will predispose you to developing a chest infection or it may even kill you. Do not take the risk of this happening.

Post-operative observations

When you have had an operation or a procedure that involves the administration of an anaesthetic or sedation, you should have your observations done at least hourly for the first four hours after your operation or procedure.

After that the rate of observations will be governed by the type of operation or procedure you have had, how sick you are after your operation, or if you are receiving patient controlled analgesia (more about this later in the section 'Advantages, disadvantages and dangers of using a PCA'). Most patients in intensive care are continuously monitored via machines.

If you have had an angiogram, make sure the nurse is checking the puncture site every half hour for the first four hours, hourly for the next four hours, and four-hourly after that until you go home. If you notice the outside of the dressing has new, fresh blood on it, or you notice blood escaping from the dressing, call your nurse immediately.

Excessive snoring or excessive swallowing

If you visit your friend or relative and they are asleep and appear to be excessively snoring or swallowing, ask for them to be turned on their side if possible and for the nurse to do their observations. These observations should include a blood oxygen saturation level. Ask for the nurse to keep on doing these observations at least every hour until your friend or relative wakes up.

This is especially important if your friend or relative is obese and/or has:

- just come back from theatre
- been given medication or taken illicit drugs that make them feel drowsy
- just eaten or drunk something
- had a head injury
- drunk any alcohol
- had a stroke
- had an operation on their face or neck.

Basic care of surgical wounds

A surgical wound should always be inspected at several key stages. The first time will be when you come out of surgery and are in recovery (you will probably not remember this happening). The next time should be by your primary nurse when you first come back from theatre, and lastly by the surgeon who did the operation if she hasn't already inspected your wound.

The important thing to remember about this wound inspection is that you should never allow anyone to lift up your dressing, remove your dressing, or touch the wound in any way without making sure they have washed their hands thoroughly. They should also wash their hands thoroughly after they have touched your dressing. If the dressing is removed or lifted up in anyway, ask your primary nurse to clean the wound and change the dressing. Do not allow the old dressing to be simply placed or taped back into position.

After the initial inspections, wound inspections and dressings will be governed by several key factors:

- the type of wound and where it is
- the type of wound dressing used, if any (some wound dressings are designed to stay on a wound for several days before they are changed, while some have no dressings)
- if the wound dressing starts to leak
- if the wound becomes infected or is slow to heal
- if there are any stitches or clips holding the wound together
- if there is a drain close to the wound.

However, if you have any concerns about your wound at all, ask for it to be reviewed. You should have someone review your wound if:

- it starts to become painful or itchy
- the wound or surrounding skin looks red, inflamed and/or is hot to touch or swollen
- the dressing starts to lift off or falls off
- the wound develops an odd smell or starts to ooze fluid

- the edges of the wound start to gape open or start to come apart.

The other aspect of wound care is your role in preventing the wound from becoming infected. This begins the day of the surgery when you will be asked to shower before your operation. You will be advised to wash with the antiseptic liquid soap hanging up in the shower. Use it. However, before you do, take some of the soap out of the dispenser and thoroughly wash the taps, the shower rail, the arms of the shower chair if you use them, and anything else with which you come into contact.

Continue to do this throughout your admission if you share these wash facilities with other patients or if additional equipment is brought into your private shower facility. This is because some patients have very poor personal hygiene habits, or are unable to adequately adhere to good personal hygiene habits, and whilst the wash facilities are cleaned on a daily basis they are not cleaned inbetween patients unless it is a private en-suite.

On leaving the shower, use a paper towel to open the door and/or wash your hands again after you have left the shower.

You have to be very vigilant about this, especially if you have any open wound or sore on your body. Try not to touch the dressing, and on no condition should you lift the dressing to touch or to look at the wound or to show it to others, unless specifically instructed by nursing staff to remove the dressing and/or wash the wound.

Getting adequate nutrition and fluids

While these are basic requirements for maintaining good health, they are even more essential when you are recovering from an illness in a hospital and when you may not have eaten for a while.

Apart from building yourself up in the pre-operative period if at all possible, consider having someone bring in, or order in, nutritious food for you to eat if you do not enjoy or find it difficult to eat the hospital food. Check with your doctor to see if there are any dietary restrictions you need to consider.

Start with nutritious soups and increase these as your appetite improves. Most wards have a fridge and microwave for use by patients, and nurses can be asked to heat up food on your behalf.

Think about having high energy, high protein snacks and drinks brought in for you. Have your food and drink labelled and stored in the communal fridge. A snack trolley comes around in most hospitals on a daily basis but these will have to be paid for by you.

If you have problems swallowing thin fluids, you will probably be assessed as requiring thickened fluids. Should this be the case, you can have thickening powder brought in for you if it is not provided by the hospital.

This will be particularly useful if the hospital only supplies limited amounts of thickened water or only supplies thickened fruit juices or cordials. You will not feel like swallowing thickened fruit juices or cordials all the time. An ability to thicken water, soup, tea and coffee will be a great help. Thickening powder can be bought from most pharmacies and can be used in consultation with your doctor.

If you have the occasion to involve yourself in helping your friend or your relative eat their food or drink their fluids, there are a few general rules to follow before you do so:

- Ask your friend's primary nurse if they can eat and drink and what form this can take if any (fluids can be thickened, restricted, clear, no milk or solids, or free fluids; while food can be such things as low-salt, low-residue, textured food, soft, diabetic and normal).

- Ask the primary nurse to sit the patient up if possible.

- Avoid using a straw for fluids.

- If your relative coughs when you are feeding them or giving them fluid, stop what you are doing and call a nurse. Do not persist with oral intake.

- Discourage the patient from talking or laughing when they are eating or drinking.

- Give them small quantities of food.

- Make sure they have finished the last mouthful before putting another one in.

- If your relative has lost sensation in any part of their mouth, encourage them to feel around the desensitised part of their mouth with their tongue to ensure no food is left there.

- Do not assume your relative can eat the food or drink the fluid that arrives for them on a food tray. A mistake could have occurred and they were not meant to receive it.

- If you are heating the food up in the microwave or making your relative hot drinks in the ward's kitchen, make sure it is not too hot. Test it on yourself.

- If you have any concerns about the amount or quality of food your relative is consuming, ask for them to be referred to a dietician, to be started on a food chart to monitor their food intake, and to be weighed on a daily or twice-weekly basis.

If your relative is given medication which makes them drowsy either just before, or during eating stop feeding them and ask the patient's primary nurse to turn them over onto their side and into the recovery position if possible. Also ask for this to happen if they are given this type of medication within 4 hours of eating. Keep them there until they are fully awake.

If you come from a culture that prohibits eating during the day at certain times of the year, and you intend to observe this practice as a patient while in hospital, consider opting for elective surgery at a later date if possible. For the most part, hospitals do not accommodate these different eating practices very well.

Getting adequate rest and sleep

With the best intentions or with little regard, wards are noisy and stressful places to be, even at night. If it isn't a patient in a neighbouring bed snoring, it is nurses talking loudly, or doctors turning on the lights to examine sick patients. I suggest you bring earplugs and an eye-mask with you into hospital and ask the nurses to be quiet at night.

Try to get some rest during the day. It is imperative you get adequate rest and sleep while you are a patient both for your physical and your psychological well-being.

If you cannot sleep, ask the nursing staff for some hot milk. Alternatively, you can ask the doctor to write you up for some sleeping medication. However, you might want to ask the doctor to prescribe you a sleeping pill other than temazepam. It is not unusual for patients who are given this drug at 10 pm to be awake by 2 or 3 am the following morning.

If this happens to you while you are an inpatient in hospital, ask the doctor to prescribe a different type of sleeping pill. What concerns me is that few prescribing doctors seem to know this about this drug. I can only conclude they do not listen to their patients and it must have been a highly effective marketing campaign.

In addition, temazepam seems to cause unsteadiness when standing for those that wake at night.

If you are prepared to supply it, doctors will often write up your favourite herbal remedy or even a tot of alcohol to help you to sleep.

Remember, sleep deprivation is used as a form of torture and it is used because it is highly effective. A lack of sleep or adequate rest it is not conducive to a quick recovery in hospital or to a heightened sense of well-being. Chronic tiredness is a great stressor on the body and will not aid your recovery.

If one of the reasons that you cannot sleep is because you are in pain, do not lie there suffering and not sleeping. Ask for some analgesia. Do not be fobbed off by a nurse saying "You are not due any analgesia", or "the doctor will not write you up for any more" or "the doctor is too busy and will not be able to come and write up the medication for you" or 'it's not time yet'.

Ask to have the doctor write up some additional analgesia. If the hospital has electronic medication charts, the doctor can access these remotely and the medication can be written up quite quickly if the doctor is too busy to attend the ward where you are. There is no reason why any patient should remain in pain for any length of time.

If the pain is muscular in origin, ask the nurse for some heat cream to be rubbed into the area. If the pain is thought to be the result of 'wind' ask the nurse for some peppermint water if you are able to drink clear fluids. Peppermint water is great for relieving wind pain and hiccups and can be given to you without a doctor's prescription.

Ensuring your continual improvement in hospital

While most people start to feel better after a few days, for others it may take longer. It is not useful to compare yourself to the other patients who have had the same operation.

How long it takes for you to feel better after an operation will depend on:

- the type of operation you have had
- your age
- how long you have been ill, before your admission to hospital
- whether you developed complications during or after surgery.

These factors will generally govern how long it will take for you to start feeling better after an operation. However, if you:

- are experiencing continual pain
- do not feel like eating

- are having trouble eating the food you are given
- are having trouble passing urine, opening your bowels, or getting yourself up and off your bed and walking

mention this to your doctor and ask for an explanation. Sometimes your recovery can feel like two steps forward and one step back, or as one patient said recently "one step forward and 12 steps back".

Do not ignore new signs and symptoms

The one thing to remember is that new or different signs and symptoms can arise once you are admitted to hospital and following your discharge home. They can be unrelated to your original presenting medical condition.

You can develop conditions:

- by virtue of being admitted to hospital
- by virtue of not receiving adequate fluids or eating a low residue diet
- following treatment with certain medications
- following bouts of inactivity like bed rest
- following the breaking of certain bones
- by simply being unlucky and developing another medical condition at the same time.

Do not assume the new signs and symptoms you develop in hospital or following your discharge home are normal, or are related to your existing or previous medical condition.

Often you will be the first one to notice if things are going wrong, such as you:

- develop pain in the back of a leg

- develop chest pain

- feel short of breath

- start feeling nauseated

- start to vomit

- stop passing urine as much as you normally do

- become constipated.

As soon as they occur, mention them to your primary nurse or to your doctor before your discharge, or to your GP or community nurse if you have been discharged home. In the case of vomiting, inform the nurse each time you vomit.

Case study

Patient B had a laparotomy, division of adhesions and a small bowel resection for a gangrenous twisted bowel.

All was going well with his post-operative recovery until the seventh day when he began to feel nauseated. Patient B told his nurse he was feeling nauseated and she gave him medication designed to relieve his nausea. It did not work. Patient B continued to feel nauseated all morning despite the medication.

By the afternoon, he had begun vomiting. He mentioned it to the nurse. She mentioned it to his treating team.

The nurse began a fluid balance chart for the patient, on which she recorded how much he was drinking, urinating, and vomiting in a vomit bag at his bedside.

Unbeknown to the nurse, however, Patient B was also vomiting when he went into the toilet to urinate. Consequently, she was unaware of just how much the patient was vomiting. As a result, the patient's fluid balance chart was inaccurate.

Based on the amount of vomit recorded on the fluid balance chart by the nurse and how many times the patient appeared to be vomiting, the patient's treating team decided to leave the patient overnight. They did not order any additional investigations or intravenous fluids. Patient B continued to vomit and became quite unwell overnight.

During the night, an abdominal x-ray was ordered for the patient. The x-ray showed Patient B had a small bowel obstruction. A nasogastric tube was inserted and Patient B was started on intravenous fluids.

The treating team would have known what was wrong with him earlier if they had known just how much he was vomiting, and treatment would have been started sooner.

Protecting children and the intellectually disabled

Any unaccompanied child or intellectually disabled person in hospital is vulnerable, and there are some people who will seek to take advantage of this vulnerability even in hospitals.

All young children should be informed not to let anyone touch their genitals without one of their parents or a female nurse being present. This education should begin before they go to hospital or while they are in hospital, and as soon as a child is old enough to recognise the different parts of their body.

If your young child or intellectually disabled person is admitted to hospital, consider staying with them throughout their admission to hospital. Do this, even if you have to ask trusted others to look after your other children at home. For some of you this will be impossible. If this is the case, insist that a female chaperone is present whenever a male health professional examines, treats, or provides any kind of intimate care for your child. This applies to both doctors and nurses.

For older children this is more problematic. They will probably not be responsive to the idea of either of their parents being present when they are intimately examined by a doctor.

In these instances, leave instructions on the child's file that any practitioner who has occasion to examine their child in a parent's absence will be required to write down in detail in the child's medical file how they conducted the examination and why. I would encourage you to maintain an open dialogue with your child about the need for such vigilance.

The same also applies to any male wardsperson who has to transport your child for a procedure or investigation, and to anyone who visits your child in hospital such as a teacher or those entrusted to offer pastoral care.

If you think I am being unnecessarily alarmist, consider these two recent case studies from the United Kingdom, and the case-study of Dr. John Rolleston who is one of the subjects of the Royal Commission into Institutional Responses to Child Sexual

Abuse's current enquiries here in Australia.

Case study

In 2014, Dr Myles Bradbury, a paediatric haematologist at Addenbrooke's Hospital in Cambridge in the United Kingdom, confessed to committing a number of sexual offences against young boys aged 8 to 17 years over a three-year period between 2009 and 2013.

Case study

The late English entertainer, Jimmy Saville, was allowed to work as a hospital porter in a number of hospitals in England at night. It is understood that he used this opportunity to sexually abuse a number of children and intellectually disabled young adults.

Case study

In 2013, Dr Rolleston was convicted of sexually assaulting a number of adolescent boys in a GP's practice and in a hospital where he worked. On each occasion the boy was separated from his parent or guardian, or had arrived at the GP's practice or hospital alone.

The boys presented for such things as a sore throat, an injured ankle, a need for a medical certificate to explain a school absence, or pain in the coccyx area following a fall.

Dr. Rolleston would sometimes perform rectal examinations on the boys, while encouraging them to masturbate themselves to the point of ejaculation. He would do so on the pretext of examining the boys' sperm for blood. At times he would masturbate the boy himself.

The Royal Commission into Institutional Responses to Child Sexual Abuse in Australia is currently conducting a number of public hearings into the way investigative bodies respond to alleged cases of child sexual abuse against health practitioners.

One of its terms of reference is as follows: "the experience of a number of patients of health care services in New South Wales who were sexually abused as children in private medical practices and public hospitals".

As part of their enquiry, the Royal Commission is hearing how the Office of the Health Care Complaints Commission (HCCC) in New South Wales responded to the men who made complaints against the Dr. Rolleston mentioned above. For more information, contact the Royal Commission's website: www.childabuseroyalcommission.gov.au

TECHNICAL INFORMATION

Intravenous lines or giving sets

Intravenous giving sets or lines are long transparent plastic tubes used for the administration of intravenous fluids and medications. They come in various shapes and have several uses. Some are designed to go through electronic pumps, others are designed to rapidly administer intravenous fluids such as blood, while others are designed to be regulated by the nurses and are disconnected after use.

Whatever the intravenous lines are used for, the rule of thumb for intravenous lines is this: If the intravenous lines are being intermittently connected on the back of other intravenous lines or are being used for the administration of total parenteral nutrition (TPN) or the administration of blood these lines should be changed every day. If they are being used solely for the administration of clear intravenous fluids, they should be changed approximately every 72 hours.

All burettes, bags, bottles or syringes that are attached to intravenous lines should be changed on a daily basis.

In addition, all intravenous lines must be anchored to your skin in some way either with some soft tape, Tubigrip®, or with a bandage. They should not be solely connected to the hub of the cannula. This is because a line that is not anchored to the skin is likely to dislodge a cannula to which it is attached. Alternatively, they can cause the skin to open up around the insertion point of the cannula making it more prone to infection.

Some wards have a practice of changing intravenous lines that are used for the administration of intravenous antibiotics every day. Some wards have a practice of changing the lines that are only used for intravenous fluids on certain days, irrespective of how long they have been up for. While this seems wasteful, it is to ensure the changing of these lines is not missed and they do not stay up for longer than they should.

Whatever is the case, each line that is put up should be labelled with the date when it is to be replaced. This should be monitored on a daily basis by your primary nurse. This is something you can also monitor as a patient.

Finally, some of the intravenous lines that can be used contain latex. If you are allergic to latex and are having intravenous fluids, remind your primary nurse about this on a daily basis and certainly before the line is used or changed.

Caring for PICC and central lines

Some people will require a PICC or a central line while they are a patient in hospital or while they are patients out in the community. PICC or central lines are designed to stay in the body over a long time. They are primarily used:

- for the administration of a number of intravenous medications

- for medications considered to be toxic to the body, such as chemotherapy

- to preserve a patient's peripheral veins

- for intravenous feeding

- for ready access to the blood of those patients who require multiple blood samples to be taken.

The only differences between a PICC and a central line is that a PICC line is peripherally inserted, and is usually inserted via an arm, and the end of a central line can terminate in the right atrium of the heart.

Things to watch out for those who have a PICC or central line are these:

- they must be inspected at least once a day

- central lines should be handled as little as possible and should be anchored to the skin so they do not become entangled

- a 10ml syringe or more should be used when accessing the line

- the nurse should not attempt to force any intravenous fluid through the line if any resistance to the flow of the fluid is encountered

- the entry point of the line should always be covered with a transparent dressing and this dressing should be changed at least twice a week

- they should always be redressed if they appear to be leaking, or the transparent dressing starts to lift off or falls off

- the roller clamp on the individual lines should always be shut when not in use and if your particular PICC line has roller clamps

- the injection ports should be changed twice a week, and the line at the discretion of the medical officer

- no one should be taking your blood pressure on the arm in which you have a PICC line inserted

- lines might be syringed with normal saline, or 'locked' with heparinised saline when not in use.

Caring for arterial lines and puncture sites

Most people who have arterial lines either have them in theatre or in the intensive care setting. They are used to take arterial blood for blood gases and/or to facilitate the arterial monitoring of sick patients. Consequently care of an arterial puncture site will probably be more concern to a relative of a patient than the patient themselves.

The two things to be mindful of where arterial lines are concerned is to ensure that: 1) the arterial line is securely held in position at all times and 2) pressure is applied to the puncture site for at least five minutes when the arterial line is removed. This should be longer if the patient is on blood thinning medication such as warfarin. Someone should also apply at least five minutes of pressure to an arterial puncture site when a medical officer has just taken a one off sample of arterial blood for blood gases. This sample is usually taken from an artery at the wrist or in the groin.

Caring for a colostomy or ileostomy

A colostomy or ileostomy is when a piece of large or small bowel is brought out onto the surface of the skin of the abdomen through which you pass faeces into a bag.

The piece of bowel that is brought to the surface (the ostomy) usually resembles a small red rosebud

An ileostomy results in you passing liquid faeces into a bag, and a colostomy results in you usually passing a formed stool into a bag. These bags are then either changed and thrown away, or emptied down the toilet.

In the immediate post-operative period, your primary nurse should be looking at the ostomy on an hourly basis and feeling its temperature through the clear plastic bag which will be covering the ostomy. Your nurse will be checking to make sure your ostomy is:

- warm to touch

- red in colour and not dusky

- raised above the surface of the skin

- not bleeding.

If your primary nurse is not doing this, ask her to do so. If you feel up to it, you can do this too.

Taking blood for cross-matching

If your doctor is of the opinion you need to have a blood transfusion, you will be asked to consent to this administration if you are able to do so, unless it is an emergency. In the event of an emergency and you are unable to consent for whatever reason, the blood will simply be given to you unless you have documentation with you prohibiting the hospital from doing so, as in the case of Jehovah Witnesses.

Each person has a particular blood type. This is either A, B, AB or O. While some people with blood types such as AB are universal recipients (they can receive blood of any blood type), other people can only receive blood of a certain blood type. To ascertain what blood type you are, a doctor or nurse will take a small sample of blood from you and send it to the pathology department for checking.

As it is important you receive blood from a compatible donor, this process has become formalised in Australia. When the doctor or the nurse has taken your blood, you will be asked to sign a form to the effect that you were the person from whom the blood was drawn. You will also be asked to check that the details such as your name, address, and date of birth on your medical labels or 'Bradmas' that are placed on the blood tubes and at the top of the pathology request, are correct.

If you are unable to bear witness to this procedure or to the accuracy of the information on the Bradmas, a (second) nurse will witness this on your behalf. However, this (second) nurse should be there during the whole time the blood is drawn from you and put into the tubes with your Bradmas on them. If she attempts to leave after the nurse or the doctor has drawn the blood, and before it has been put into the tubes, ask her to stay until after this process has been completed.

Apart from bearing witness to the cross-matching process, the only other things you have to bear in mind when receiving a blood transfusion are as follows:

- Make sure two people check the information on the label that has been affixed to the outside of the bag of blood, and they do this against the information on the accompanying blood form and the details printed on your identity band. You should be able to hear them read out your name, date of birth, your hospital number, the serial number of the bag of blood, the expiry date of the bag of blood, and your blood group if you are familiar with it.

- When you look at the bag of blood you should be able to see that it is a dark red in colour and not green.

- The blood should be cold to touch.

- Before the blood transfusion is started, the nurse should take your observations. As a minimum, the nurse should do your observations 15 minutes later and after the transfusion has been completed. Some hospitals require nurses to continue to do a patient's observations every 30 minutes during the entire time the blood is being infused.

- When the nurses bring the bag of blood to your bed it should be started immediately. It should not be allowed to hang by your bed or sit on your bedside table for any length of time without being started.

- The transfusion should be completed within three to four hours.

- When the blood has been given, the line should be flushed with normal saline to flush all of the blood out of the line and into your vein.

- If at any time during the blood infusion you develop a headache, chest pain, pain in your back, or start to feel unwell, feverish or nauseated, call the nurse immediately and ask for the transfusion to be momentarily stopped while she does your observations.

- Unless you are actively bleeding, and if possible, seek to have yourself reviewed by a medical officer before the administration of a second unit of blood and check to see if its administration is really necessary.

Elevating the head of the bed

Some types of surgery require you to have the head of the bed elevated during your immediate post-operative period. How long this is continued for will depend on the type and extent of the surgery you have had.

Sometimes you will wake up from your anaesthetic to find you are sat up with the head of the bed elevated. If this is the case, do not lower the head of the bed or ask anyone to do this for you. Keep your head elevated until advised to do otherwise by your primary nurse.

Protecting your health following urinary catheterisation

A urinary catheter is a transparent plastic tube that is passed up the urethra into the bladder. People are normally catheterised with a urinary catheter if:

- they cannot pass urine

- they have had gynaecological, lower abdominal, or orthopaedic surgery on their hip or pelvis

- there is a need to monitor a patient's urinary output

- they require bladder irrigation

- they require to have a sample of urine to be sent to pathology quickly.

If the plan is to catheterise you with a urinary catheter and you know you have just started a new drug or suspect you may have a pre-existing urinary tract infection, inform the nurse who is about to catheterise you before she starts.

A urinary tract infection is often characterised by an urge to pass small and frequent amounts of urine and can produce a burning sensation when you urinate. Your urine often smells and can be dark in colour if you have an infection.

A prophylactic dose of an antibiotic can be given to you before you are catheterised or consideration can be given to not catheterising you at all.

Should you need to be catheterised, there are a few things you should be mindful of. Whenever anything is put into your body there is an increased risk of developing an infection.

Just as this is true with the insertion of intravenous catheters, so it is with urinary catheters.

What makes urinary catheters so problematic for patients is that they are put into the bladder.

While urine is ordinarily sterile, it contains substances which facilitate the easy growth of organisms. Thus the bladder is an environment which is very conducive to the growth of infections. Organisms can grow quickly in urine and can become very harmful to patients when grown in urine in the bladder.

Urinary catheters are especially problematic for women. This is because they are inserted in the bladder via the urethra, which for women is close to the anus or bottom. This necessarily increases the risk that organisms from the bowel will ascend up the catheter and into the bladder.

With this in mind, here are a few tips for reducing your risk of developing a urinary tract infection following urinary catheterisation:

- If there is time, wash your genitals with hospital supplied liquid soap and dry yourself well with the inside of a freshly laundered hospital towel before being catheterised.

- Drink plenty of water after you are catheterised, unless you are on restricted fluids.

- Have the catheter removed as soon as possible.

- Wash your hands before and after touching any part of the catheter, or the entry point of the catheter in the body.

- Avoid wearing knickers or underpants while you are catheterised.

- If the tubing is disconnected from the catheter, ensure the nurse swabs both ends of the catheter and the tubing with antiseptic solution before they are reconnected.

- Have the catheter changed in accordance with the manufacturer's instructions (usually four to six weeks after the date of insertion).

- Have the drainage bag changed every week.

- Clean the point where the catheter enters the body and the tubing itself well with hospital liquid soap each time you shower, and dry yourself with the inside of a newly laundered hospital towel.

- Wipe your bottom from front to back if you are a woman. Never wipe your bottom forward onto the catheter.

- Ensure the catheter bag is hanging from the bed or lying on a bluey (pad with blue plastic coating). Try to avoid having the catheter bag lying on the floor.

- If the urine looks cloudy or starts to smell, have the nurse take a specimen from the catheter tubing and have it sent to the pathology department for testing. Do not allow the specimen to be collected from the drainage bag.

Other things to be mindful of when being catheterised with a urinary catheter are:

- Make sure the catheter is securely fastened to your leg.

- For men, check to make sure the catheter is not held too tightly against one side of the urethral opening of the penis so making this area of the penis red, inflamed and/or sore.

- If the catheter stops draining, in that there is little or no urine in the catheter bag, have your primary nurse perform a bladder scan to see if the catheter is blocked.

- If the catheter becomes painful for whatever reason, insist your primary nurse checks the catheter and attempts to solve the problem. A catheter is not normally painful.

- If you are mobile, ask the nurse to change the drainage bag to a leg bag. This can then be strapped to your leg and will make it safer for you to mobilise.

- Seek to have your nurse perform a urinalysis on a specimen of urine from the drainage bag every few days. This will ensure any developing urinary tract infection will be identified and quickly dealt with.

If you are advised it is thought you have a urinary tract infection while you are catheterised and a sample of urine is collected from the catheter, seek to find out the results of the test from the second day.

Keep making enquires on a daily basis until you are informed of the result. If you have developed an infection and you haven't already started on some antibiotics, seek to have these started as soon as possible.

If you need to be catheterised over a long period of time or indefinitely, consider consenting to the insertion of a suprapubic catheter if offered to you. This will be easier for you to manage and will reduce the risk of you contracting a urinary tract infection.

Advantages, disadvantages and dangers of using PCAs

One of the big changes that has occurred in health has been the introduction of patient controlled analgesia (PCA). This is an intravenous analgesia drug administration system which is controlled by the patient. The analgesia is delivered to the patient via an intravenous PCA pump through an intravenous line.

The patient controls the amount of analgesia they receive within pre-set limits through the use of a button. The pre-set limits are set by an anaesthetist and changes to this delivery system can only be initiated by an anaesthetist. The analgesia in the pump can make you feel euphoric and drowsy.

> What is important about this system is that the patient has to be able to press the button themselves and should do so when in pain. This ensures the patient is conscious enough to press the button and cannot give themselves an overdose.

You will be obliged to have oxygen while using a PCA. This will generally be delivered via nasal prongs. These prongs will continuously deliver approximately two litres of oxygen to you for the duration you on the PCA. This oxygen may be increased if it is necessary to do so.

While the oxygen can cause drying of the nasal passages which can be uncomfortable for you at times, do not take them off. You need the oxygen. This is because the type of medication you will be receiving through the PCA can affect your ability to breathe deeply. This in turn may result in you having a reduced amount of oxygen in your blood stream which can make you confused at times.

If the drying of the nasal passages is a problem for you, ask your nurse for some moisturising cream rather than taking off the nasal prongs.

There is a specific regime that should be followed when using a

PCA. This is as follows:

- Under no circumstance should you allow a relative, a friend, a nurse or a doctor to press the PCA button on your behalf.

- Press the button when you are in pain.

- On no condition should you be given or should you take any other strong analgesia while you are on a PCA, unless this has been prescribed for you by an anaesthetist. This includes Panadeine® and Panadeine® forte.

- A nurse should check your level of consciousness, count your respirations, take your pulse, do your blood pressure, check the saturation of oxygen in your blood and check how much medication you have received via the pump every hour for the first six hours you are on the PCA. The nurse should do this every two hours for the next 18 hours and thereafter every four hours for the entire time you are on the PCA. If your primary nurse is not doing this, ask for this to be done.

For those of you have a friend or relative on a PCA, be aware that this medication can make them feel very drowsy. They can be so drowsy they are at risk of choking on their food or fluids if they are lying down on their back.

If you intend helping your friend or relative to have a drink or to eat their food while they are on a PCA and drowsy, seek help from the nursing staff to sit them up before you start. Only do this after you have found out from the nursing staff if they can sit up, and if they can eat and drink.

An underwater sealed chest drain

Occasionally a patient has to have an underwater sealed drain inserted through their chest wall and into their lung cavity.

A chest drain is used to drain air, blood or fluid out from around the lungs into a drainage bottle or bag. This will enable the lungs to re-expand properly, enabling you to breathe more easily.

The underwater seal prevents air or fluid re-entering the chest.

The things to watch out for with underwater sealed chest drains are these:

- Make sure your call button is within easy reach at all times.

- Ensure that, once your drain is inserted, your primary nurse does your observations every 15 minutes for the first hour, hourly for the next four hours, and then four-hourly during the whole time the chest drain is inserted.

- If you suddenly become short of breath or have trouble breathing, call the nurse immediately.

- Make sure your primary nurse records the amount of fluid in your drainage bottle or bag every hour, and replaces the drainage bag or bottle when it is three-quarters full.

- Have adequate analgesia to allow you to breathe deeply.

- Make sure the health professional washes their hands before touching your drain or tubing, unless it is in an emergency.

- Make sure at the start of each shift your primary nurse checks the dressing covering the entry of the drain through your chest wall and where the drain is connected to the tubing of the bag or bottle.

- Make sure the drainage tubing is anchored to your skin in some way.

- If the drain stops draining, or you notice your drain is suddenly leaking more blood or fluid than normal, call the nurse immediately.

- Do not sit on the tubing or allow it to become kinked in anyway.

- If the drain becomes disconnected from the tubing, call the nurse immediately.

- Do not try and get out of bed or out of your chair for the first time with a chest drain in place without the help of nursing staff.

- If the nurse is of the opinion that you can walk with your drain, or you are transferred to another part of the hospital on your bed with a drain, make sure the drainage bag or bottle is below the level of your chest at all times and is kept upright.

- If you are unsteady on your legs or you walk with a walking aid, do not attempt to walk with your drain.

Having a tracheostomy

A tracheostomy is a surgical opening in the anterior wall of the trachea in the neck through which a tube is passed to facilitate breathing.

The tube enables the air we breathe to enter the trachea and lungs directly, thus bypassing the pharynx and larynx. A tracheostomy also bypasses the upper airway of the mouth and nose where the air is normally warmed, filtered and moistened.

The type of tube you have inserted will depend on why you are having a tracheostomy, how long it is to remain in place, if you can swallow, and how you are to be nursed after insertion.

There are a few things to be mindful of when you have a tracheostomy:

- Make sure your call button is within easy reach at all times.

- If you have any trouble breathing when you have a tracheostomy in place, press down on your call button immediately and continuously and indicate to another patient to call out for your primary nurse immediately.

- If you have what is called a 'cuffed' tube, make sure at the start of each shift your primary nurse sucks the tube out before checking the pressure in the cuff.

- Make sure your primary nurse checks the dressing and the ties holding the tube in place on a daily basis, and that she replaces these if they become soiled or if the dressing leaks.

- If you have a mask covering the end of the tracheostomy, especially if it is delivering oxygen to you, do not remove that mask.

- Ask your nurse to wash your mask(s) every day.

- If the sputum or secretions you are coughing up out of your tube become difficult to cough up or become sticky, indicate for the nurse to give you a normal saline nebuliser.

- Ensure the nurse does not try to use the suction catheter on more than one occasion when suctioning your tube, unless of course it is an emergency.

- Make sure the nurse washes her hands before putting on gloves to suction your tube, unless of course it is an emergency.

- Make sure your suction catheter is in easy reach for suctioning out any secretions in your mouth.

- Do not use the thick ended suction catheter to suck out the opening of your tracheostomy tube, unless it is an emergency. Use a clean tissue each time.

- Make sure the nurse rinses the suction tubing out with fresh water after each successful suction.

- If you are coughing up any blood or your sputum becomes streaked with blood or becomes yellow or green, show the nurse the sputum and have her inform your treating team.

- Drink plenty of fluids if allowed to do so and attend to regular mouth hygiene.

- Keep your hands clean.

Nasogastric tubes

As the name implies, a nasogastric tube is a tube passed via the nose into the stomach. Nasogastric tubes are used for one of three reasons:

- to feed a patient with liquid food

- to rest the gut by removing fluid generated by the stomach

- to remove stomach contents in the event of the ingestion of toxic substances.

They generally come in two sizes. A thin bore white nasogastric tube is used to feed patients and a large bore transparent nasogastric tube is used to drain or aspirate stomach contents.

The things to watch out for with a nasogastric tube:

- Do not allow anyone to put anything but air down your tube without first checking its position in your stomach. This should be done with a chest x-ray or by listening for air entry via a stethoscope below the level of your left ribs.

- If you start coughing or you feel breathless at any time when you have a nasogastric tube in place and you are receiving nasogastric feeds, call your nurse immediately and bend the tube in half to block the flow of the feed.

- If your nasogastric tube is accidentally pulled up and is then pushed down again, ensure the position of the tube is rechecked before anything is put down the tube.

- Any feeding bags connected to your nasogastric tube should be replaced every 24 hours and the nasogastric tube should be changed monthly.

- If a thin bore feeding nasogastric tube is not in use at any time, make sure the nurse maintains its patency by syringing it with water once a shift. Sometimes this water needs to be sterile.

- If your medications are to be given down your nasogastric tube, make sure these are crushed finely and mixed well with water, and your tube is flushed with water before and after they are given.

- If there is no fluid coming up the nasogastric tube, and especially if you are becoming nauseated, encourage the nursing staff to put air down the tube first before trying to aspirate the stomach contents. Sometimes an air lock can prevent the aspiration or drainage of stomach contents up and out of the tube.

- If you are having your nasogastric tube aspirated, ensure this is done at least four-hourly and more frequently if there is a lot of fluid coming up the tube.

- If blood comes up the tube, have yourself reviewed by a medical officer.

- Ensure your nasogastric tube is securely taped to your nose and to your cheek. This will prevent it from being inadvertently pulled out.

Neurovascular observations

Should you incur an injury to a limb, be it a broken bone or significant injury to the tissues of your limb, or you have a skin graft, ensure the nurses are doing what are called neurovascular observations. These should include checking to ensure:

- you can feel the outer extremities of the limb and that this sensation feels normal to you

- your limb is warm

- your limb has a good pulse

- your limb is the same colour as the other limb

- you can move your fingers or toes as appropriate

- you have good capillary return to your limb, in that when the skin is pressed and then released blood returns within 3 seconds

- your limb is not too swollen.

If your limb starts going cold or blue, the sensation in your limb changes, the pain increases, or you cannot move your limb, ask to have your limb reviewed by a medical officer.

WHAT TO DO IF THINGS GO PEAR-SHAPED

Ideally much of what has been discussed so far will do much to protect you as a patient during your admission and your eventual discharge home. However, mistakes will occur and will continue to occur in the future.

If you have any concerns about your treatment or the actions or inactions of one of the staff members, there are things you can do about it. These I have outlined below.

What it means to 'stay between the flags'

For the most part, patients display early warning signs when their condition is deteriorating. These warning signs often occur long before their condition becomes critical.

These early warning signs usually involve adverse changes to a patient's observations. These can involve a patient's respiratory rate, pulse, blood pressure, temperature, blood oxygen saturation levels, blood sugar level, Glasgow Coma Scale (GCS), and/or urine output level.

On the basis that only one person has ever died in Australia while swimming between the flags on beaches that employ life-guards, the Clinical Excellence Commission of New South Wales has adopted the image of keeping patients within the flags when conceptualising a set of safe parameters for patients.

The idea is you try and keep a patient's observations within a defined set of parameters or flags, and escalate their level of care should their observations fall outside these parameters.

This escalation involves calling a medical officer and often instituting additional immediate care such as administering oxygen. It always involves increasing the number of times a patient's observations are taken.

In NSW, parameters considered to be 'normal' for adults have been formally set as follows:

- respiratory rate between 10–25 breaths per minute
- blood saturation level >95%
- pulse or heart rate between 50 and 120 beats per minute
- systolic blood pressure (upper level) <180 and >100, and diastolic blood pressure (lower level) <90
- temperature above 35.5 and below 38.5
- blood sugar >3mmols and <20 mmols
- >100mls of urine in a four-hour period via an indwelling urinary catheter (IDC)
- <200mls of urine for 2 hours via an IDC.

If an adult patient's observations fall outside these parameters in NSW, or there are changes to a patient's Glasgow Coma Scale (GCS), a health professional must activate the 'Clinical Emergency Response System' (CERS).What form this takes depends on how far outside these defined parameters a patient's observations has fallen.

While most patients' observations normally lie within these parameters, others do not. For instance, some elite athletes have resting pulse rates below 50 and some people's normal systolic blood pressure can be less than 100. I for one, have a normal blood pressure of 90/50, which for others would be very low.

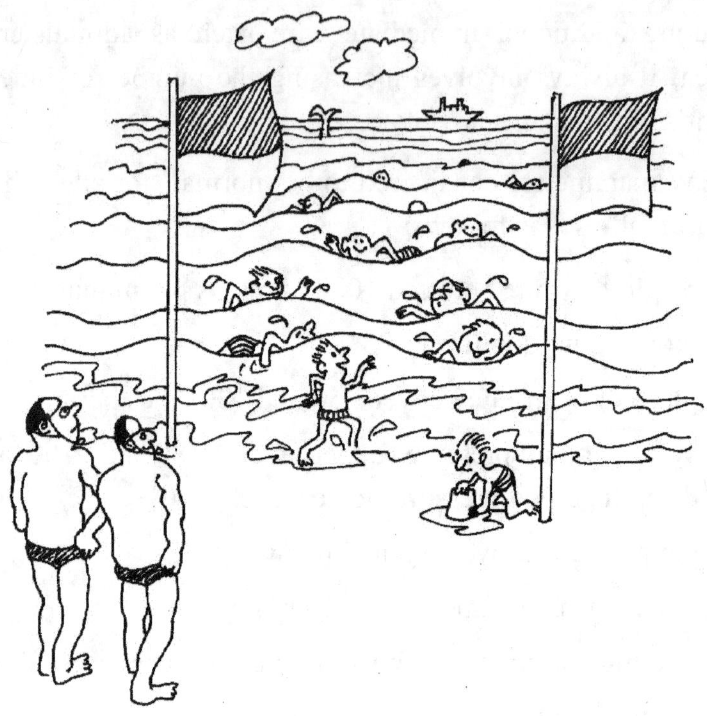

A patient's blood saturation level can often be quite low first thing in the morning, especially if they are woken from a deep sleep. The saturation level normally rises when they are sat up and after they have taken some deep breaths.

For respiratory conditions such as chronic obstructive pulmonary disease (COPD), a normal blood oxygen saturation level is usually between 85–90 percent and can be as low as 80 percent. As a result, revisions are made to a patient's 'calling criteria' for an escalation of care given the individual differences of the patient. However, changes to a patient's calling criteria can only be made by a medical officer and must be reviewed every 72 hours.

What is considered normal for a patient will usually be based on:

- their observations on admission, if they are admitted as an elective patient
- pre-existing medical conditions
- what is currently wrong with them
- what they say is normal for them
- what has happened to them while they have been a patient.

If the hospital to which you are admitted does not employ such a system to protect their patients, you might want to insist they adopt the New South Wales system for you during your admission.

For this to be effective, you need to know what observations are normal for you, and to ask the nurse who performs your observations to tell you the results. If you find any of your observations fall outside these defined flags at any time, you can ask to be reviewed by a doctor.

Going on up the line

There is much you can do if you have tried to raise your concerns about what is happening to you and when no one seems to be listening or acting on your concerns. There is a designated level of seniority for nurses and doctors in hospitals.

For nurses it is:

1. Your primary nurse

2. Nurse-in-charge of the ward

3. Nurse Unit Manager (9am–4pm on weekdays) or 'After-hours Manager' at all other times

4. Director of Nursing or General Manager.

For doctors it is:

1. Junior medical officer

2. Registrar or senior on wards (after hours)

3. Specialist or consultant

4. Medical Administrator.

Keep going on up the line until you have some kind of satisfactory resolution to your concern.

Patient advocates

If you do not feel able to address your concerns yourself, ask a friend, relative or legal representative to talk or advocate on your behalf. Anyone can act as an advocate. You just have to be able to trust this person will accurately and diligently represent your views, and stick up for you should the need arise.

Do this on your own behalf or on behalf of others. This is especially true for people who:

- are elderly

- are young and inexperienced

- become mentally unwell at times

- have an intellectual disability

- live in out-of-home settings

- are from a CaLD background and have no one who can speak up for them.

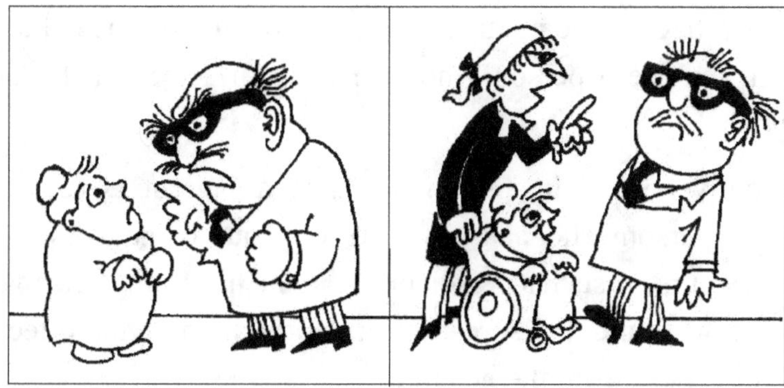

For those who become mentally unwell at times or become incompetent at making their own decisions, you need to appoint this person in the presence of a legal representative when you are well and considered competent to do so.

You should legally empower this advocate to be:

- able to access any information about your medical condition

- an active participant in any medical decision regarding your treatment

- able to obtain a second opinion for you when you are unwell

- able to represent your views at a mental health tribunal or guardianship tribunal

- your legal guardian when you are unwell, or deemed to be incompetent or incapable of making your own decisions by your treatment team or others.

You should also empower this person to be able to seek a second opinion on your behalf even if your treatment team deems you competent and capable of making your own decisions regarding your health care. Do not under-estimate the importance of doing this if you are a person who suffers from a mental illness at times.

Alternatively, the hospital may have a patient advocate or support person who can advocate on your behalf. Ask your primary nurse if such a person exists in the hospital. If the matter involves the potential spread of infection, involve the infection control officer from the hospital.

Avoid weekend problems

If you have any concerns about your recovery by Friday, do not wait until the weekend to raise your concerns. This is because your specialist does not work on weekends unless she is rostered on to work the weekend. In addition, even if your specialist is in the hospital at this time, she will only be in the hospital to treat patients presenting as emergencies. She will not ordinarily be available to address any of your concerns, unless you are the emergency.

On weekends your care will be left in the hands of a junior doctor. This doctor may be inexperienced and unfamiliar with the type of treatment you have received, and may be slow to recognise when things are going wrong for you as a patient.

In addition, this doctor will be reluctant to make any major decisions regarding your care themselves and will be reluctant to disturb your specialist at home on the weekend. They will also have limited shared access to more senior staff.

Therefore, do not delay. Raise your concerns as soon as they occur and do not wait for the weekend.

It's never too late to start raising your concerns

While you may have delayed raising your concerns initially, it is never too late to start.

Do not delay raising your concerns further because you feel silly for not having raised them sooner, and do not try to hide how long this has been a problem for you. Delaying still further may only compound the problem. It may make dealing with the problem more difficult.

Chapter 3:
Discharge from hospital

PROTECTING YOURSELF LEADING UP TO AND AFTER YOUR DISCHARGE

Planning for your discharge from hospital

Planning for your eventual discharge from hospital should begin on admission and long before you are discharged home. While for the most part people feel better when they leave hospital, some people can feel the same or even worse when they are discharged home. It takes time to recover from any hospital admission.

How long it takes to recover from an operation will depend on a number of things:

- the extent and length of time you have been sick for in the lead-up to your admission

- how old you are

- if you have any pre-existing illnesses or medical conditions

- the type of operation or treatment you have had

- the length of time you have spent in hospital

- when you were last in hospital

- if you have been left with any kind of incapacity

- whether you had any complications or setbacks

- the amount of rest and nutrition you have had while you have been in hospital.

These will generally govern how long it will take for you to feel better and to recover from your admission.

If you know, or suspect you are going to be left with some kind of incapacity when you are discharged from hospital, either on a temporary, long-term or permanent basis, you will need some kind of home assessment before your discharge. This will be arranged by the hospital's occupational therapist.

Be honest about what you feel you are going to be able to manage to do for yourself. Do not be pressured into thinking you can do more than you can physically and safely manage to do.

Care arrangements should be organised for dependants and pets. The hospital's social worker and home care support services should be organised to help you with these long in advance of your discharge.

You may need modifications to your home and car. Planning for these should begin as soon as it is deemed necessary. Some modifications such as the installation of ramps may need local government or housing department approval in advance.

Respite care and Rehabilitation

For the most part you will need to be looked after when you are discharged home. Friends or relatives should be primed to start preparing for this in advance. With pressure on hospital beds being what it is, the decision to discharge you from hospital will often be made long before you are fully recovered and before you are psychologically ready to be discharged. You will often need some ongoing support when you go home. Be realistic with what you can do. This is the time to be assertive.

If you do not think you will be able to cope at home and have no one to look after you when you are discharged home, and especially if you are the primary carer for someone else, ask to go to respite care or rehabilitation (rehab), and for the person you care for to go into respite care with you. If you are a pensioner in Australia, you can currently go into respite care for 63 days a year.

Alternatively, find out if the hospital offers a transitional care service which can provide you with care in your own home. If they do, ask to be referred to this service.

Rehab is not the same as going into a nursing home. It is solely geared to preparing you to go home if that is where you want to go. Do not think that if you go to into respite care or rehab it will mean you will never get home. Going to rehab until you feel better often makes the difference to your perceived and actual ability to return home.

In addition, do not assume that 'going to rehab' means we think you have a drug problem. There are different types of rehab.

Do not let yourself be discharged before you are ready

The best way to protect yourself in the lead-up to your discharge from hospital is to refuse to be discharged home until you are ready to look after yourself, or until you have arranged for someone to look after you. One patient negotiated a delay to her discharge until after her daughter had arrived from overseas. This was a month after the hospital had deemed her well enough to go home.

If your doctor is of the opinion you are ready to be discharged and you or your family member does not think this is the case, ask her this question: "What would you expect me to be able to do before I am ready to be discharged?" If her answer does not accord with what you can do in reality, decline to be discharged until alternative care arrangements can be made.

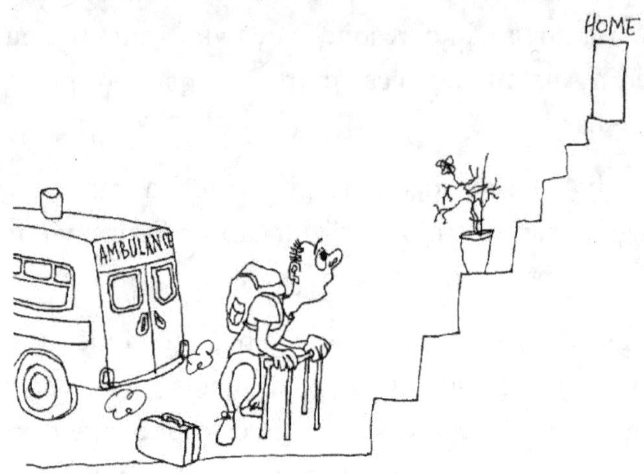

Restoring home services

If you had the services of a community nurse or home care before your admission to hospital, it is highly likely you will need these services on your discharge. Make sure these services have been restored for you before leaving the hospital. Find out when this service will restart.

If you will need medical supplies on discharge, and the hospital's plan is to discharge you on Friday, make sure the hospital provides you with adequate supplies to see you over the weekend until further supplies can be organised for you by a community nurse.

The discharge letter

When you are discharged from hospital you will be given a discharge letter addressed to your nominated GP. This letter will have been written by a junior doctor who has been asked to organise your discharge.

If you have occasion to leave the hospital before the discharge letter has been written, it will be sent on to your GP. If you do not have a GP, inform the nursing staff before you leave so it can be sent on to you.

The discharge letter is an important part of your discharge process.

The discharge letter informs your GP:

- that you have attended the emergency department or were admitted to hospital

- of the care you received in the hospital

- of any complications that arose during your admission

- the follow-up care you require if any

- of any proposed changes to your medication regime.

If you are discharged home from the emergency department or the hospital and you have not been given a discharge letter to give to your GP, follow up with your GP to make sure they have received the letter.

If your GP has not received the follow-up letter, ask them to call the emergency department or the specialist's receptionist and ensure this is sent.

Checking your discharge medications or prescription

When you are discharged from public hospitals and some private hospitals you may need to have some medications.

Often you will be given some medications to tide you over until you can see your GP for a prescription or until you can have your hospital prescription filled by your local pharmacy. These medications are issued from the hospital's pharmacy for you after they receive a prescription from the ward doctor who discharges you from hospital.

If you are discharged home on a Friday afternoon, and you have not been given any medications to take over the weekend and it is too late to fill your prescription, ask the hospital to supply you with these medications.

In my opinion, providing discharge medications for patients is one of the most important yet poorly managed parts of the hospital discharge process. It is poorly managed for three very important reasons:

1. The process is handled by no less than five different people, and sometimes six or more.
2. Discharge often happens quickly and with little pre-planning.
3. Discharge often occurs before 10am in Australia. This is one of the busiest times of the day on the ward.

The people involved in the prescribing, dispensing and supply of your medications are:

- your specialist
- the doctor who writes up your discharge medications

- the pharmacist who makes up the prescription and supplies the medications

- the nurse or wardsperson who collects your medications from the pharmacy

- the nurse who gives you your discharge medications

- your designated carer who collects your medications or you the patient who takes the medications.

In my experience as a senior investigator with the Office of the Health Care Complaints Commission, the more people involved in what should otherwise be a standardised process the greater the chance a mistake will occur.

Case study

My 90-year-old Aunt was recently discharged from hospital where she had been admitted for a flare-up of a pre-existing medical condition.

Unbeknown to her, the specialist's plan had been to prescribe her oral antibiotics for 10 days following her discharge home.

On her discharge, the hospital did not supply her with antibiotics, did not provide her with a prescription, and more importantly did not advise her she needed to be on the antibiotics. They did not advise her daughter who arrived to collect her either.

The antibiotics were only recommenced two days after she was discharged home by her GP, when she again started displaying symptoms, and after the GP had made enquiries of the hospital.

If you are a competent person you can offset the chances of any risks occurring with your discharge medications by doing several important and fundamental things.

> Quick guide to taking medications home on discharge
>
> - Take only the medications you brought with you to hospital.
>
> - Take only medications dispensed for you by the hospital pharmacy.
>
> - Take only the same medications at the same doses prescribed for you when you were admitted to hospital.
>
> - Do not take those supplied for your use while in hospital.

If your medications are kept in the drawer of your bedside locker and you are allowed to go through this drawer to collect these medications yourself, check that the medications you are taking home are the ones you brought with you into hospital and that the doctor still wants you to take these medications following your discharge home.

Do not be tempted to take those supplied by the hospital for your use in hospital and which will also be in the drawer. Do not do this irrespective of how tempting this may be to you.

In addition, some nurses think they are being generous towards you and give you all of the medications stored in the drawer of your bedside locker. They do this in the mistaken belief they are doing you a favour by helping you to save money. While their motive is admirable, this practice is fraught with danger and should not happen. This is because the medication in your bedside locker:

- may have been dispensed for the patient who previously occupied your bed and may have been inadvertently left in your drawer by mistake

- may have been put back in the wrong box

- may have been dispensed in a different dose and/or in a different form to that which you have been taking at home

- will not have the administering information printed on the outside of the box.

Make sure that any new medications that you are taking home with you, have been dispensed for you by the hospital's pharmacy.

Make sure they have a label affixed on the outside of the box on which your name, MRN, date of birth, and the administration instructions for the medication are printed. If this is not the case, do not take these medications home with you.

Secondly, make sure you are discharged home on the same medications and the same doses that were prescribed for you when you were admitted to hospital, unless of course your doctor does not want you to take these medications anymore. If medications have been ceased, medications have been added, or their doses have been changed for any reason, ask for an explanation from the doctor who has prescribed your discharge medications.

Just because certain medications are given to you in hospital does not necessarily mean you should be taking them when you go home. A mistake could have occurred. Be particularly wary if you are given narcotic medication to take home with you, especially if you have not been taking this medication in the lead-up to your discharge. If you are in any doubt, check this with your discharge nurse or make an early appointment with your GP and discuss this with her.

Case study

A nurse was asked to give two patients their discharge medications. On review of the medications, she noticed that oxycodone had been dispensed for both patients.

Oxycodone (commonly known as Endone®) is a very strong narcotic medication. The patients were prescribed this drug in a dose range of 5–10mg, every six hours, for when needed (PRN).

Having looked after both patients that day, the nurse knew that neither of them had complained of pain in the lead-up to their discharge and to her knowledge had not been given oxycodone during the previous shift.

Instead of giving the patients their prescribed medications and discharging them home, the nurse delayed the discharge of the two patients and rang the doctor who had prescribed the medication.

She asked him why he had prescribed this drug for these patients. The doctor confirmed what she had suspected. He had simply prescribed all the medication that had ever been prescribed for the patient on their medication chart.

He had done this instead of checking to see if the patient had been receiving the drug in the lead-up to their discharge and whether they still needed to be taking the drug following their discharge.

Neither of these patients had been receiving this drug in the lead-up to their discharge and one of these patients had not had the drug during her entire admission.

Be extremely wary of taking medication such as oxycodone, OxyContin®, morphine or Panadeine® Forte when you are discharged home, unless you are also prescribed medication that counter-acts the effect of these drugs. This is because this type of medication slows down the bowel. Consequently, it can make you very constipated, very quickly at times.

This is particularly important for the elderly, for the disabled who have mobility problems, for those who do not drink very much or are on restricted fluids, and for those who eat low residue diets or have gut motility problems.

If you have been taking antibiotics in hospital, check to see if you should be taking these antibiotics following your discharge home. This is especially important if you have been having intravenous antibiotics in the lead-up to your discharge.

If any of your newly prescribed medications make you feel sick, do not just stop taking the medication without first talking this over with your GP and your pharmacist. Sometimes your pharmacist can suggest and your GP can prescribe, a different version of the same drug, or alternatively prescribe you another drug that will counter the negative effects of the first drug.

Keeping yourself safe post-discharge

As previously mentioned, a number of patients are discharged home long before they are ready to be so. Often they are still in pain and are not as mobile as they used to be. This can put people at risk of developing a number of complications as a result of this pain and/or resulting immobility when they are at home. These complications can arise from:

- not being able to cough properly and clear secretions from the respiratory tract
- a tendency to reduce the amount of fluid they consume so as to decrease the number of times they have to get up to go to the toilet
- a reduction in the overall level of mobility and agility
- resting in bed or in a chair for long periods of time.

And as a result they can develop other complications. If you are finding you are in pain or have decreased mobility when you get home, inform your GP at the earliest opportunity.

For anyone who has had been admitted to hospital for any length of time, they will usually be emotionally exhausted, may well be under nourished, and may be chronically sleep deprived. It is important you look after yourself or have someone to look after you following your discharge home.

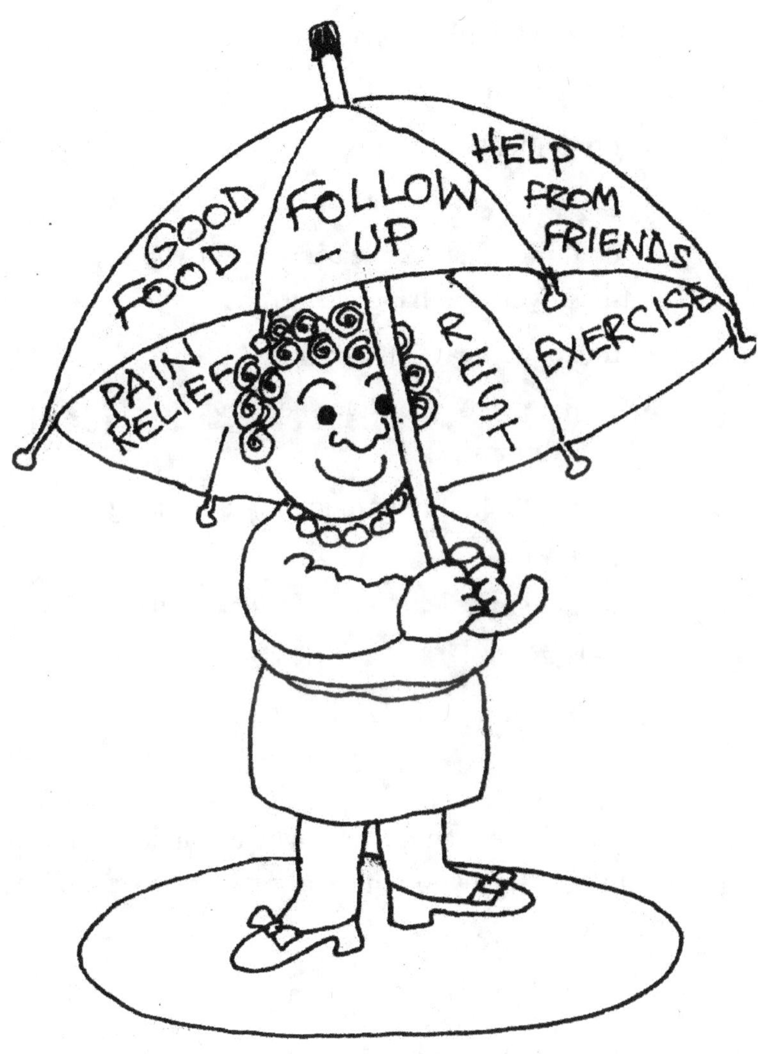

Don't underestimate how low you can feel following discharge.

When you get home:

- eat nourishing meals

- drink plenty of fluids

- get adequate rest and sleep

- do things that are pleasurable for you and make you feel happy

- do not do heavy housework

- do not make extensive shopping expeditions

- do not look after grandchildren for long periods

- do not struggle to meet the demands of others.

You can expect to feel quite low when you leave hospital, irrespective of how well you felt in hospital. This state of mood will often be worse if you:

- felt down before your admission

- were in hospital for a long period of time

- had any other adverse event happen to you while a patient in hospital

- were admitted to intensive care

- were in pain for long periods of time

- felt you were not getting better at anytime

- had anything go wrong with your surgery

- had a surgical procedure

- had an anaesthetic

- had little rest or sleep

- had long periods when you were not allowed to eat and lost weight

- have been put on certain medications

- have little perceived, or actual, support when you do go home.

This is normal. Do not under-estimate how low you can feel on discharge from hospital.

Do not be hard on yourself. This is a time to be gentle with yourself and to expect the same from others.

If your low mood persists, or seems to be getting worse, make an appointment to see your GP as soon as you can. Do not allow yourself to get so low you do not feel like calling your GP.

Attending for follow-up

If the specialist wants you to attend for follow-up after your discharge home, go. This is especially important if she needs to give you some results or if there were are any complications arising from the surgery you had.

Attending for follow-up is an important part of the process of protecting yourself as a patient. If you do not plan to attend for follow-up, let the specialist's receptionist know so your appointment can be allocated to another patient. Be advised, though, if you do not attend for follow-up your specialist is under no obligation to contact you irrespective of your results.

If the reason you do not intend going for follow-up is due to anticipated financial hardship, call the specialist's receptionist and let her know. Try to negotiate a reduced fee or to be bulk-billed. It is always worth trying. Most specialists went into medicine with a genuine desire to help and look after people and not to simply feather their own nest. They will often surprise you with their benevolence, irrespective of how they may have treated you as a patient in hospital.

If, however, you do not go to see the specialist for any reason, make arrangements to see your GP instead.

Chapter 4:
Protecting yourself and others in the future

PROTECTING YOURSELF

The best way to protect yourself is to avoid becoming a patient in the first place, and from becoming a patient again in the future. You can help to do this by taking steps to protect your health.

While we all know we can protect our health by eating sensibly and healthily, reducing the amount we drink and smoke, avoiding illicit drugs, wearing a seat belt or a safety helmet, getting plenty of rest and exercise, maintaining a good weight, engaging in safe sex and reducing the amount of stress in our lives, there are other ways we can protect our health. Outlined below are some other strategies you may not have thought of. I am interested to hear of others for the next edition of this book.

Medications can make you feel sick or have no therapeutic benefit

All medications have to be chemically altered or metabolised by the body into their metabolites to have either a beneficial effect on the body or to be excreted from the body in urine by the kidneys or in faeces through the bowel.

The cytochrome P-450 enzymes in the body are responsible for 75 percent of all drug metabolism. While the metabolism of drugs primarily occurs in the liver, some metabolic processes occur in the kidneys, in the gut wall, in the lungs, and in the blood plasma.

While some drugs require specific enzymes to be metabolised by the body, other drugs can be broken down or metabolised by a number of different enzymes.

In addition, some drugs or food can induce enzyme activity, while other drugs and food can suppress enzyme activity. This then makes it more likely a person will either have adverse side-effects from the medication or derive no therapeutic benefit from the medication at all. In addition, as people age so enzymatic activity decreases. This means older people often need smaller doses of the same drug for their medication to be effective.

The other factor to consider is that, just as we have genetic variations that govern individual differences with regard to our skin colour, height and facial features, so we have individual genetic differences that govern the functioning and effectiveness of our cytochromes. This is important when you consider most doctors use the 'Monthly Index of Medical Specialities' (MIMS) as a guide when prescribing medications for their patients.

According to Associate Professor Les Sheffield in Australia, MIMS recommended drug dosages are based on an ideal of patients being extensive metabolisers of drugs. Unfortunately, this is true for only 50 percent of the population. Other people are poor or ultra-rapid metabolisers of drugs.

Consequently, a number of people prescribed drugs are either receiving:

- too much of the drug
- too little of the drug, or

- the wrong drug

for the drug to have any therapeutic benefit.

Consider this when taking drugs that are important to you such as anti-depressants, anti-psychotic, chemotherapy or analgesic drugs, when taking a number of drugs, when taking drugs with adverse or toxic side-effects, and when taking drugs with small therapeutic windows.

According to the coroner in Victoria, Australia prescription drugs were involved in 82 percent of overdose deaths, and this is increasing rapidly.

You do not want to:

- be prescribed any drugs for which you have ineffective cytochrome P-450 enzymes

- be prescribed a number of drugs that all require the same cytochrome P-450 enzyme to be bioactivated or broken down

- be prescribed drugs for one condition that can inactivate enzymes required to bioactivate or breakdown drugs prescribed for a second condition

- consume excessive amounts of a drug such as alcohol and sugar in its various forms that can affect the ability of organs such as the liver to manufacture these enzymes

- drink grapefruit juice that can inactivate one of the most important cytochrome enzymes, CYP3A4

- take Saint John's Wort that can affect certain important cytochromes

- take a number of medications if you have pre-existing liver or kidney damage.

Consequently, learning about your individual cytochrome enzymes through simple pharmacogenomic testing can have significant benefits for you if you need to take medications. This testing can identify gene variants which can help predict which patients will endure adverse side-effects to which medications, and which patients will derive no benefit from medications prescribed for them.

I would strongly recommend pharmacogenomic testing for those patients who:

- do not respond to certain medications

- experience any adverse or toxic side-effects to medications

- take, or are about to take, such medications as warfarin, clopidogrel or tamoxifen

- are on a number of different medications

- have a family history of medication problems or adverse reactions to medications

- take medications known to be toxic to the body such as chemotherapy and human immunodeficiency virus (HIV) medications

- are scheduled under a mental health act and who are made to take their medications

- are elderly and on newly prescribed medications, and who suddenly develop delirium with no identifiable cause.

This will at least ensure you have cytochrome enzymes that can effectively use and breakdown the therapeutic metabolites of the drugs prescribed for you.

Pharmacogenomic testing can be facilitated for you through several online companies, either by taking a painless scraping of the cells on the inside of your cheek or via a simple blood test.

Have a health plan

If you have a chronic illness such as asthma or epilepsy, you might want to adopt a health plan to protect yourself, and to inform others as to the best way they can help you. Health plans, such as an Asthma Action Plan, can be downloaded from Asthma Australia www.asthmasaustralia.org.au.

Health plans, such as the one below, can show people how they can best help you in the event you have a fit or seizure. Such a plan would involve people:

- protecting your head from injury
- watching to see you are breathing
- removing tight clothing from around your neck
- staying with you until the seizure has passed
- rolling you onto your side when the seizure has stopped, and checking to make sure there is no food or vomit in your mouth
- watching to see what happens to you so they can accurately describe the seizure (for instance, how long you were twitching, if you wet yourself)
- calling an ambulance.

Do not have anyone:

- put anything in your mouth
- attempt to restrain you

- move you unless you are in danger.

Co-opting other government or private agencies

Many elderly and disabled people are now being looked after in their own homes by government funded or private 'home care' services. For many people, this involves having people come into their home to help them to shower two or three times a week.

This may be the only time anyone sees them naked, unless they become ill. You would think this would be an ideal time for people from this agency to review their client and comment on what they find to their client, or to their client's next-of-kin with the client's permission. This doesn't always happen.

Last year I stayed with my elderly Aunt on the occasion of her 90th birthday celebrations in Perth. While I was there, I helped her shower. When my Aunt was undressed, I noticed a large black mole on her left buttock. I brought it to her attention. She advised me that she hadn't known it was there.

When I spoke to her daughter and my cousin about the mole, she advised me that she had only noticed the mole herself when she had taken her mother to her GP for her vitamin B injection. My Aunt's GP had looked at the mole and advised my cousin it was nothing to worry about. My cousin also confirmed what I had already suspected – no one from my Aunt's home care service had informed her about the mole and no one had referenced it in her home care history.

The mole is large and certainly worthy of mention and could easily have been malignant. When I reviewed the documented history maintained by the agency workers, there was no space to record any such observations the agency staff could have made of their clients.

In my opinion, this represents a missed opportunity for primary health care. It also serves as a warning to both the elderly person receiving home care services and to their relatives. Do not rely on staff from the home care services to inform you or your relatives if they notice anything wrong with you. If you are a relative of such a person, and if they agree, consider undertaking this care yourself on an ad hoc basis. This way you can monitor the overall health of your relative.

Not only should you be checking their bodies for any new lumps and bumps or the growth or change to moles, you should also consider weighing them on a regular basis to make sure they are not losing weight. This is especially important for relatives who are becoming forgetful or have difficulty managing for themselves.

Give these home care agencies written permission for their staff to contact your next-of-kin or your GP on your behalf should they notice anything wrong with you. They will need written permission from you to enable them to do this.

Avoiding certain occupations or work practices

If possible, avoid or limit your exposure to professions or to certain workplace practices that expose you to harm or injury. This may entail factoring in ways to offset this harm in other areas of your life or taking active preventive measures to prevent this harm. For instance, dentists have the highest rate of suicide of any professional group so they should potentially look to limiting stress in other areas of their life.

Other examples are check-out operators and baristas who experience high rates of repetitive strain injuries (RSI) to their shoulders and arms, and workers in heavy industry who should wear safety equipment to protect their eyes, ears, hands and feet.

Look after your teeth and gums

Tooth decay and gum disease can lead to significant health problems if allowed to develop and remain untreated. It is thought that the body's ongoing exposure to the type of bacteria that live deep in the pockets in your gums and possibly in the cavities in teeth that form as a result of tooth and gum disease, can cause conditions such as heart disease, Type 2 diabetes and cancer (The Guardian 20 July 2015).

This is why it is so important to brush your teeth properly on at least a daily basis, but twice a day if possible (I recognise that some of you will be dependent on others to clean your teeth for you). This is especially important if you eat a high carbohydrate diet, drink sweetened drinks and juice on a regular basis, already have these conditions, or have a compromised immune system.

Ideally you should brush your teeth with an electric toothbrush that has an oscillating head, use a fluoride based toothpaste containing an anti-bacterial agent, and go to a dentist and dental hygienist on an annual basis. You should also allow your children to drink fluoride enriched tap water, and limit the amount of soft drink and juice that you and they consume.

While I know that going to see a dentist is very expensive, especially for those on low incomes and benefits, please refrain from do-it-yourself dentistry such as filling your own teeth, popping your own dental abscesses and extracting your own teeth.

Lastly, if you are going to use an anti-snoring device, it is important that you brush your teeth properly, clean the device properly with soap and water with a brush, and douse the device in an oral anti-bacterial solution before you insert it.

Using a medication dosette box

A dosette box is a plastic box divided up into compartments in which you can store your medications. Each section is labelled vertically under the day of the week and horizontally under the time of day in which you store your medications in accordance with your GP's instructions and the pharmacy's administration guidelines. A dosette box is a way of physically ordering your tablets so you have a visual reminder of which tablet to take and when.

As soon as you cannot remember if you have taken your medication or not is the time to start using a dosette box. You should do this irrespective of how old you are. This is because some medications such as Parkinson's medications are time critical, in that they have to be taken within 15 minutes of a set time. Others such as the anti-rejection medications I have already mentioned need to be taken every day.

Pick a day when you are relaxed and not too busy to fill the dosette box for the week, and check it every night before you go to bed to ensure you have taken your pills. Leave a note for yourself by your toothbrush if necessary.

Taking breaks from lengthy computer games

A number of people now play or involve themselves in computer games. This often means sitting at a computer for hours at a time. Sometimes they are so engrossed in these games they do not drink adequate amounts of fluids or get up and move on a regular basis.

I know how bad this can be because I once sat at a computer for 7½ hours without moving while playing the addictive computer game 'Lemmings'.

Unfortunately, this activity poses a significance risk to its participants. This is primarily because they are at an increased risk of developing a DVT (deep vein thrombosis) or blood clot in the deep veins in the leg.

If this embolus or blood clot breaks off and travels through the vein and into your lungs, this will become a pulmonary embolus. This is a serious event. If the blood clot is large enough it can block the blood flow to the lungs and can cause sudden death. This risk is increased if the participant is overweight or has had a DVT in the past.

If you are a person who engages in this activity, you might want to consider wearing support tights, ensuring you have plenty of fluids to hand while you are playing the games, and setting an alarm to go off at regular intervals to remind you to drink and to get up and walk around.

Not buying breast milk from unregulated sources

Some people have taken to buying breast milk from unregulated sources online. These people include parents or carers of infants, cancer sufferers, bodybuilders, and adult fetishists who want to be fed as babies from a baby's bottle.

While breast milk is the best thing to feed a small infant, it has not been found to offer any advantage for body builders or cancer sufferers. And certainly, feeding anyone breast milk from unregulated sources such as those obtained online has not.

Researchers from the University of London's school of

medicine and dentistry have been so alarmed by what they found when researching the practice of buying online breast milk they have just written an editorial piece for the British Medical Journal before their study has been completed. In one study they looked at, 90 percent of the breast milk was contaminated with bacteria. In another they found breast milk was being sourced from intravenous drug users, greatly increasing the risk that these online supplies of unscreened breast milk will be contaminated with HIV, hepatitis and syphilis. Other samples had been found to be adulterated with water and cow's milk.

Not having cosmetic surgery performed by unregulated and untrained practitioners

An increasing number of cosmetic procedures such as the injection of Botox, the insertion of fillers, and eyelid surgery are being done in backyard parlours and beauty salons by untrained, inexperienced and unregistered practitioners such as beauticians.

They are doing this because there is a demand from people who feel they cannot afford to have it performed by a plastic surgeon, or performed by a nurse under the supervision of a plastic surgeon. Consequently, this puts people at greater risk of severe infections, nerve damage and facial disfigurement.

Not only is the insertion of Botox or fillers by an unregistered practitioner illegal in Australia, these beauticians are:

- generally sourcing their product via the internet from unknown suppliers
- potentially using unsterile and inappropriate instruments.

There is no way of verifying if the products they are using are safe, they cannot be tested for their quality, and there is no way of knowing if they are being injected correctly or safely. Consequently, people are at risk of contracting life-threatening infections or suffering permanent facial disfigurement. Given this, I would strongly urge you not to engage in these practices with such people.

In addition, cosmetic surgery is not a recognised speciality in Australia. Any doctor can set themselves up as a cosmetic surgeon. A GP can be a cosmetic surgeon and cosmetic surgery requires no additional training.

Plastic surgeons go through years of training. This is why plastic surgery is expensive. If you think your physical appearance is important enough for you to consider going through painful surgery to have it surgically enhanced, it is worth paying for it to be done by a plastic surgeon.

Not having ultrasound scans performed by untrained or unregistered practitioners

An anomaly currently exists in Australia whereby any Tom, Dick, Harry or Rawinia can purchase an ultrasound scanner and perform ultrasound scans at home. There is no current legal requirement for them to be a trained, accredited or registered sonographer in Australia.

Case study

Ms Rawinia Hayes was fined A$6,000 plus court costs this year, when she pleaded guilty to six charges of accepting payment but failing to supply goods or services in breach of the Australian Consumer Law.

She was not charged under the Crimes Act or under any health practitioner Act.

Ms Hayes had passed off dozens of fake ultrasound images of unborn babies to pregnant women.

Therefore, I would recommend that if you are going to have an ultrasound scan performed that you check that the person who is going to perform your ultrasound scan is registered as an accredited medical sonographer. Check the Australian Sonographer Accreditation Registry to make sure: www.asar.com/directory

Illicit intravenous drug users

A word of warning to intravenous drug users. If you damage your veins with illicit drug use, as you often do, you will have few peripheral veins left for nurses and doctors to cannulate when you become sick. Consequently, you will have to be much more vigilant to protect those veins you still have.

If a suitable peripheral vein cannot be found, you are going to need the insertion of a central line for the administration of intravenous medications and fluids. This is a much more invasive procedure and carries more risks.

Using home medical equipment

An increasing number of people are using medical equipment in the home. This equipment can vary from medical alert buttons, peritoneal dialysis equipment, portable home oxygen units, to CPAP machines to facilitate breathing at night.

While this is revolutionising care in the home, it doesn't come without its difficulties and needs adequate planning. For instance, all these machines require electricity to function, and while some have batteries with which they can operate in the event of a power outage, others do not.

Therefore if you are going to use such a system at home, you are going to have to plan what you are going to do in an emergency when power to the home is cut-off, and may not be reconnected for days. This may vary from visiting a public building to re-charge the battery, to having a petrol operated generator to run the machine. In addition, all these medical devices should be connected to an anti-surge protector to ensure they are not damaged when power is restored.

Knowing your extended family medical history

If you do not know your extended family medical history, try and find out. This is especially important if:

- there is a history of early deaths or major medical illnesses in the family
- you originate from, or belong to a culture in which close family members tend to inter-marry.

If you have had family members who have had early deaths, consider accessing their death certificates if possible, or alternatively accessing genealogy information about them on websites such as www.ancestry.com.au . This can be a valuable source of information. For instance, I have been able to find out there is familial history of early deaths from breast cancer on my late father's side of the family and, while it seems limited to his great aunts and their families at the moment, this may well prove to be of relevance to me and my niece in the future. It is a family history I have shared with my GP and with my extended family members on my father's side of the family.

Sharing your extended family medical history

While it is important to find out your extended family medical history, it is just as important to share your medical history with your GP and with your extended family. This is especially true if you are having treatment for a major medical illness that has a genetic basis, if you have any allergies, if you have ever had a life-threatening reaction to certain medications, or you have relatives who have, or who have been successfully treated for, the same condition.

This enables your GP to assess your risk factors for developing certain diseases or illnesses, to consider alternative treatment strategies, and to plan your treatment. It allows your extended kin to consider having genetic testing, and to know they too could suffer from these allergies or be susceptible to these adverse events.

This has been invaluable for me. For instance, my brother found out he is severely allergic to contrast medium when he had an anaphylactic shock, collapsed, and nearly died during an investigation. Consequently, when I have investigations involving a contrast medium I am prepared in advance for these procedures. The technicians use a more expensive, but low allergenic contrast medium and I am given medications that reduce my response to these potential allergens.

If you start to talk about what you know about your extended familial medical history to your immediate family and your relatives, you will learn more. Things you may not have known, or things you may have forgotten or have been confused about, will come to light. This will only help to protect you all in the future.

Participating in local falls prevention programs

It is estimated one in three people over the age of 65 will fall at least once a year. In response, many local health authorities have been setting up specific falls prevention programs for the elderly. They are designed to give people practical advice and suggest strategies to enable them to keep themselves safe around the house and outside in the community. They offer advice on:

- the safe use of medications
- the use of walking aids and the properties of safe footwear
- problems that arise with people's vision as they age
- how to improve the safety of your environment
- the importance of adequate nutrition and fluids
- the type of exercises designed to build strength and improve balance.

If you are over 65, I would strongly urge you to participate in these classes.

Self-learning

Carers groups, online support groups and specific talks at local hospitals can provide useful information to enable you to protect yourself and others.

Learning from others who have the same disease, illness, or health problem, and who are potentially taking the same medications as you, will often be the most useful and reliable sources of information. These are just a few examples of organisations that could be helpful to you:

- www.coeliac.org.au

- www.asthamaustralia.org.au

- www.mcgrathfoundation.com.au

If you belong to a group that has identified specific gaps in their health knowledge, or who want answers to specific collective health problems, you can have someone from your local community health centre or hospital come out to address your group and provide you with this information. If your members are from a CaLD background, seek to have them bring an interpreter with them.

Avoiding benevolent general practitioners

Your GP is in a very powerful position as far as your health and general well-being are concerned, especially if you live alone and receive home visits. While what I am about to write is controversial, I can assure you that from my professional experience with the HCCC it requires saying.

Consider doing the following with regard to home or nursing home visits by GPs:

- Consider not making your GP a beneficiary of your will. If you do make him a beneficiary of your will, on no condition should you tell him he is.

- If you want to reward your GP after your death, consider funding a training course or a piece of medical equipment at the local medical centre or hospital in his name, rather than organising to leave him money directly.

- If your doctor suggests you start having vitamin B or pain killing injections, consider only having them in the presence of a neighbour or a friend who can stay with you for 30 minutes after the injection. If you do not have a neighbour or friend who can sit with you for 30 minutes, and you need to have a vitamin B injection or a pain killing injection, consider only having it in the GP's surgery and in the presence of a friend or the GP's practice nurse.

- If your GP asks to take blood from you, consider only agreeing to do so in his surgery and in the presence of a friend or his practice nurse.

- Remember, your GP is not your friend. He is a professional person and you should treat him as such. Do not call him silly names like 'my boyfriend'. Call him by his title instead.

- If your GP visits you in your nursing or care home and wants to give you an injection or take some blood from you, ask for this to be done in the presence of one of the nurses from the nursing home.

- Have it documented in your medical or nursing care plan that, in the event you are found unconscious for any reason, you are only to be taken to a public hospital and not to a private hospital. Have it be known you are to have a full blood and toxicology test on arrival and are not to be treated by your GP if you are taken to a private hospital. Have this be known by your GP in the presence of others.

- In the event of your unexpected or unexplained death, or you die without gaining consciousness, have it be known by your GP in the presence of others that you are to have a full blood and toxicology test before your death is certified, and that this is to be done by a medical officer other than your GP.

If you think I am being unduly alarmist, be aware that a GP in Britain, Dr Harold Shipman, was able to kill most of his patients by injecting them with a lethal dose of diamorphine. He was able to do this on the pretext of taking blood from them for a medical study.

It is estimated Dr Shipman killed at least 215 of his patients over a 12-year period between 1975 and 1998, and killed nearly all of these people in their own home. He also killed some of these people in his surgery. Dr. Shipman was seemingly not motivated by financial reward when he killed most of his patients and he remains Britain's worst serial killer.

Advantages of speaking English

Many of you in Australia are from CaLD backgrounds and have not had the opportunity to learn English.

Many of you are new arrivals to this country, have been working two jobs, or have been at home raising children and have not had an opportunity to learn English. A significant number of you have not had an education, have received little education, or have been poorly educated in your own language(s) and would have difficulty learning English. Consequently, you will be at a distinct disadvantage when seeking care as a patient in an English speaking health system.

If you are an English-speaking relative, friend or even a neighbour of someone who cannot speak English, it is important you consider going with them to the GP or to the hospital when they seek treatment as a patient, if it is appropriate for you to do so. Alternatively, you can provide means by which they can be more easily understood in hospital. This may mean making yourself constantly available on a mobile phone to answer questions and provide translating services, to providing a translating application on a smartphone or a translation package on an electronic tablet.

The smartphone application I find most useful is 'iTranslate Voice translator & dictionary', which currently retails for A$6.49 from the App store. This application can translate your language into English and vice versa.

Alternatively, you can have basic words and phrases with simple pictures and their English equivalents, written down for your relative's use when you are not there.

Unfortunately, if you are not able to speak English in an English-speaking health system you are likely to be largely excluded from the decision-making process involving your own health care.

Often your nominated or self-nominated next of kin will be considered to be your spokesperson. Their views as to what is appropriate for you, or what they think you would like with regard to your own health care will often prevail.

These relatives may not respect or necessarily act in your best interests and may not accurately represent your views.

Often they are asked to translate the information the doctor wants to convey to you, rather than being asked to translate questions you want to ask of the doctor. The people who translate for you might be very selective as to the information they do translate for you.

Quick guide to the disadvantages of not knowing English

- You are likely to be largely excluded from the decision-making process involving your own health.

- Little will be explained and expected of you, and certain treatment options will not be offered to you.

- Relatives who translate for you may not necessarily act in your best interests and may not accurately represent your views.

- Instructions for procedures for medical investigations will be in English. If you do not follow these instructions the procedure may not be successful.

- You run the risk of not being understood by the English speaking health professionals looking after you, and this may result in you being inadequately or wrongly treated.

Case study

Patient C, a 92-year-old CaLD woman was admitted to hospital with metastatic cancer. This was causing a blockage to the flow of bile from her liver. As a result of this blockage, she was becoming very jaundiced. The jaundice made her skin itch and contributed to her nausea. As the toxins built up in her body, Patient C began to vomit.

Patient C did not have any pain, but she felt awful most of the time. The nausea and vomiting affected her ability to sleep and she no longer felt like eating or drinking. Consequently, a decision was made to start intravenous fluids while a decision was being made as to whether treatment should be continued or not.

As Patient C could not understand or speak English very well, her daughter was asked her view.

The patient's daughter was adamant that, despite her mother's age and diagnosis, she should receive ongoing clinical reviews and resuscitative measures should her condition deteriorate, even though it quickly became apparent her mother's condition was inoperable and terminal.

Reading Patient C's clinical notes, it became clear that at no time was the services of an interpreter employed to adequately explore the patient's views and wishes, and her daughter had been the only family member consulted.

Over the two nights I looked after Patient C, she expressed a clear desire to be able to die in English. She said "I want to die, let me die" on at least two separate occasions. I documented this in her clinical progress notes.

When I last saw this patient she was receiving intensive treatment for septic shock, which involved being given large amounts of intravenous fluids and antibiotics. She was also having blood tests.

I was asked to catheterise her with a urinary catheter with which to measure her urinary output.

The patient's daughter's views had prevailed, and while the accommodation of the daughter's views and wishes stopped short of having Patient C admitted to intensive care, she had not been allowed to die as had been her expressed wish.

If you have been in the country for any number of years and cannot speak any English, it may be wrongly assumed you are incapable of doing so. Consequently, little will be explained and expected of you and certain treatment options will simply not be offered to you.

This is especially true of procedures that require you to give informed consent. For instance, if you are having a heart attack or a stroke as a result of a blockage in your blood vessel caused by a clot, and you cannot inform the doctor if you have had any unusual bleeding such as bright red blood in your stools, black sticky stools or any abnormal bruising on your body, you may not be offered a certain drug designed to reduce the clot in your blood vessel.

This is because this drug can cause additional bleeding in your body and could pose an additional unacceptable risk for you if you have a tendency to bleed or if you are bleeding.

This may result in you not being offered this medication at all, which may result in your stroke or heart attack being inadequately treated. The ensuing damage could potentially be much worse or even fatal.

Before having a number of investigations, you will be asked to prepare for these at home and often long before you present to hospital. The instructions for these procedures will be written in English.

If you do not follow these instructions the procedure may not be successful. You may also be at increased risk of an adverse event occurring either during or immediately after the procedure. In addition, if the hospital staff are not convinced you have followed the instructions correctly and it is important for you to have done so, they may cancel or at least delay your investigation.

What you also don't want to see happen is that an understandable outburst of anger in your native tongue directed at the health professional looking after you, is misinterpreted as indicating an exacerbation of your illness if you are mentally unwell, or evidence of a delirium if you are an elderly person with an infection. This may lead to you being unnecessarily sedated just because you cannot be understood.

While interpreters can be available to be booked under some circumstances, in some situations there is simply no time. In other situations, there is a lack of motivation on behalf of health workers to engage the services of an interpreter even if they are available.

They may even be reluctant to wait until a family member can come in to translate on their behalf. This should not be so, but this is what often happens.

As demand for interpreting services increases, and governments look for ways to cut health expenditure, it is unlikely these services will be extended in the future, and may even be cut.

If you intend staying in this country and anticipate being patients here one day, try to learn English.

Not only is it important to learn English but it is just as important to practise speaking it. This is because people often revert back to speaking only languages they are most familiar with when they become sick. If you are not familiar with speaking English, you are not likely to do so when you are ill. As a result, you will not be readily understood by the English speaking health professionals looking after you, and this will often come at a time when they have little time to do so.

You will be much safer, and importantly will feel safer in an English-speaking health system if you can speak and understand English. This is not a time for things to be lost in translation.

As part of this learning exercise, you might want to watch medical drama series such as 'Doc Martin' or 'Grey's Anatomy' or reality shows that feature hospital environments. Not only will this enable you to familiarise yourself with the technical language of the hospital environment, but it will give you an insight in to how these environments work.

Australian reality programs you should consider watching are 'Kings Cross ER: St Vincent's Hospital', '24 hours in

Emergency' and 'Outback ER'. Other countries screen similar programs.

If you or your relatives do not speak English and you need the help of an interpreter, it is important you know both the language and the dialect in which you speak. Failing this, it will help if you at least know the English names for the country and region of your country from which you come. This will help to ensure the interpreter will be able to speak in both your language and in your dialect. However, there are more than 200 different languages and many more dialects spoken in Australia, and there are simply not enough health interpreters to cater for every patient who needs one.

PROTECTING OTHERS

Protecting your relatives in out-of-home care

If you suspect your relative or friend is not receiving adequate food or fluids in the place where they are living, there are several things you can do:

- Ask them how much food they are receiving and what they are being given to eat.

- Attend at meal-times and check to see if they can feed themselves and if they can eat the food they have been given.

- Check to see if they can give themselves adequate fluids and, if they can't, ask what provision is being made to ensure this is happening.

- If your relative is reducing the amount they are drinking because they are becoming incontinent, make sure they are supplied with incontinence pads and these are changed on a regular basis.

- Have it documented in their care plan they are to be weighed on a weekly basis, and offered fluids on a two to three hourly basis. This should be increased if your relative becomes sick or it is summer time.

- Make sure your relative has a regular GP and she visits on a regular basis.

- Have the GP do blood tests on a regular basis, or when necessary, to make sure your relative is being adequately fed and hydrated.

Showing support and appreciation for nurses

Nurses are generally over-worked, underpaid and largely unappreciated. This is by those who employ them, by governments who fund and regulate them, by their professional managers and colleagues who staff the wards, and by the very people they are assigned to look after. In my 20 years of experience as a registered nurse and senior health investigator this has worsened over time.

When I first started as a nurse, patients or their relatives demonstrated their appreciation of what nurses did for them. They did this by buying boxes of chocolates or baskets of fruit or giving them bouquets of flowers. This is rarely the case now.

While some patients or their relatives may occasional send a card, many do not. They often leave the ward with no expression of appreciation for what the nurses have done for them. It is now common to receive little acknowledgement, little respect and no thanks or praise for the work nurses do.

When this is coupled with the anti-social hours and the poorly maintained and under-resourced environments in which they work, life as a nurse can be very difficult at times.

Show your appreciation and respect for the nurses who look after you by asking their name and thanking them for what they do for you, and by at least trying to help yourself as much as you can as a patient.

Case study

> *In one hospital ward-based study, of the six things considered as being 'positives' at work, nursing staff named receiving 'compliments' about their work practices as being one of them. One nurse mentioned being given a pot plant by the relatives of one of the patients she had looked after.*

Actively support nurses politically by writing to your local member and to the Prime Minister directly should any government even consider reducing penalty rates for night, after-hours or weekend hours worked by nurses. Nurses are an essential and integral part of our health system, and their rates of pay should reflect this.

Not treating hospital staff badly

For a significant number of patients, I would like to take the opportunity of this book to remind them that most hospitals in Australia have a 'zero policy' to threatened or actual violence towards their staff. With this in mind, I would like to make special mention of nurses who often bear the brunt of this violence.

Some patients still need to be reminded that nurses are not domestic servants. They do not respond well to being treated badly. They do not like being given orders, being shouted or sworn at, or being talked down to. They do not like being belittled, ignored, and held responsible for things they have not done. They also do not like being asked to do things patients can easily do for themselves. Lastly, they do not appreciate being threatened, racially vilified, physically assaulted, sexually harassed and sexually assaulted, and yet these things are happening to nurses on a daily basis in some hospitals.

If some patients continue to treat nurses in this way, they will only have themselves to blame if hospitals have trouble employing and retaining nurses. They will only have themselves to blame if they do not receive the care they need, if nurses tend to ignore and distance themselves from them, if nurses won't find clean clothes for them to go home in or find them temporary accommodation in which to recover.

They will only have themselves to blame if nurses delay giving them analgesia until they are in pain, avoid them, or refuse to treat them as a patient. And finally, they will only have themselves to blame if nurses organise for these patients to be prematurely discharged from the hospital and long before they are ready to be discharged home, or worse still have them arrested, charged and carted off to the nearest police station.

This is a patient's choice, and I would strongly advise them to choose wisely least they alienate themselves from the hospital staff and unnecessarily compromise their care and treatment as a patient.

If you are a patient or a visitor to hospital and hear someone treating a member of staff badly, consider seeking help on the staff member's behalf if you are able to do so.

Making a complaint

If you have any concerns about the way a health professional is medically treating you, raise your concerns immediately or soon after it has occurred. If you feel unable to speak to the health practitioner concerned, ask to speak to the nurse unit manager. If you are concerned about a general practitioner, ask to speak to the practice manager if there is one.

If your concern is of a sexual nature, in that the practitioner has made inappropriate comments to you or has touched you in an intimate manner you feel is inappropriate or unnecessary considering your presenting medical condition, always make a complaint. And always make this complaint in writing to a health regulatory body.

- If you have been treated in Australia, you can make a complaint to the Australian Health Practitioners Regulation Agency (AHPRA), unless the incident occurred in New South Wales or Queensland. AHPRA's phone number is 1300 419 495 or you can visit their website www.aphra.gov.au.

- If the incident occurred in NSW, contact the Health Care Complaints Commission on 1800 043 159 or via their website: www.hccc.nsw.gov.au.

- If the incident occurred in Queensland, contact the Office of the Health Ombudsman on 133646 or via their website: www.oho.qld.gov.au.

Make a complaint even if you think something may not come of it, or you think it will be 'his word against mine'. This may be true, but if you complain he will think twice before doing it to anyone else. He may already have been made the subject of another complaint of a similar nature and your complaint will allow the investigative body to take action. If you don't do it for yourself, think about the next patient coming along.

If you have been treated in other countries, contact your local health authority and ask how you can make a complaint.

Protecting Medicare

When you have finished seeing a GP in Australia, and before you leave the medical practice, the GP's receptionist will ask you to sign a Medicare claim form for any consultation higher than an 'A' consultation. To reiterate, a level A consultation is taken by Medicare to indicate you have seen the GP for less than five minutes, while a level B consultation is taken by Medicare to mean you have seen the doctor for a minimum of five minutes and less than 20 minutes.

When you sign the GP's Medicare claim form, you enable the GP to make a claim for this consultation from Medicare. I have found, in some bulk billing practices I have frequented in the past, I have been asked to sign for a minimum of a level B consultation irrespective of how long I had been with the GP.

As I only tend to see a bulk billing GP for a prescription or for a medical certificate, I am usually in with the GP for less than five minutes. Consequently, this visit should only be billed as a level A consultation.

To protect Medicare and prevent health costs from spiralling out of control, refuse to sign for a level B consultation if you see a

GP for less than five minutes. If you sign for a level B or even a level C consultation when it should be a level A consultation, you are actively participating in the GP's defrauding of Medicare.

The government is aware some GPs defraud Medicare in this way. Instead of seeking to prevent this from happening, they have instead made it easier for this to occur. The Medicare website contains no information as to which item numbers pertain to which level of consultation. For instance, there is no way of easily knowing that item number '003' is a level A consultation or that '023' is a level B consultation.

I would urge you to undertake your own surveillance of GPs by doing these three basic things:

1. Register online with 'myGov' and link your Medicare number to your account. This way you can check what item number your GP has charged Medicare.

2. Record the time you entered the GP's consulting room and the time you left. If this is under five minutes, do not sign for a level B consultation.

3. If you are asked to sign for a level B or more consultation when you have only been in the GP's surgery for less than five minutes, refuse to do so and report this to Medicare.

If we do not act to prevent Medicare fraud, the government will do other things to reign in these costs. In my experience, they will do this rather than taking the more politically sensitive and challenging course of controlling these fraudulent GPs.

An example of this occurred in 2014. The coalition federal government in Australia attempted to introduce a $7 direct co-payment for visits to the GP, out-of-hospital pathology, and diagnostic imaging services. They did so on the understanding that many patients see GPs when they are not really sick. By introducing a $7 direct co-payment they sought to address this problem. They thought that if patients had to pay a $7 direct co-payment to see their GP, they would be less likely to go to their GP unless they were really sick.

The trouble with this reasoning is that some people on no income or on low incomes cannot afford this co-payment, whatever form it takes. They will either receive no medical care or they will have to go to the hospital's emergency department for treatment. This is especially true of young people who cannot claim benefits, and for those with a family member with a chronic illness such as a child with asthma. Such children will miss out on having their asthma properly monitored and treated.

Once introduced, these co-payments will invariably continue to increase over time and will ultimately affect us all. If you want Medicare to survive as an institution you have to play your part in defending it.

If you are a person who goes to their GP because you are unhappy and lonely and have no one to talk to, stop. Not only could you pick up unnecessary infections from doctors' surgeries that can make you very unwell or can even kill you, a GP's time is valuable.

A GP's time is valuable not only for their other patients but for society at large. If you and others take up your GP's appointments when you are not really sick, the costs of Medicare will continue to spiral out of control. In addition, someone who is really sick will have to wait. Consequently, you might unwittingly contribute to their ongoing ill-health or even risk endangering their life.

This also applies to calling an ambulance. Do not call an ambulance unless you are ill and need to go to hospital for emergency treatment. Some people call an ambulance in the mistaken belief that if they go to hospital in an ambulance they will be seen quicker. THIS IS NOT THE CASE. Everyone is assessed and prioritised in the same way, irrespective of how they arrive at the hospital.

In addition, the ambulance service is not a taxi service and should not be treated as such. If you call an ambulance when you do not need one, there will not be an ambulance for someone who does.

Do not put the health system at risk for yourself and for others in the future by going to see your GP or by calling an ambulance when you do not need to.

Protecting medical insurance companies

I do not have medical insurance and I do not agree people should have access to different types of health care just because they have an ability to pay. I do recognise that private health insurance companies will continue to play a role within the health system and should not be fraudulently exploited by unscrupulous hospital administrators, doctors or dentists.

If you have private health insurance, you can support this sector by doing one simple but important and effective thing: do not sign for treatment or procedures you have not had, in exchange for reducing the potential out-of-pocket expenses for the ones you have had. If everyone does this the medical insurance fees will rise, medical insurance companies will go under, and you simply won't have private health insurance to buy.

Consider boycotting any health practitioner who asks you to do this, and consider reporting them to your health insurance company, to the police, and to their registration board.

Learning from other systems of care

Case study

The old National Health System

I began my training as a registered a nurse in the National Health System (NHS) in England in the late 1970s. At the time, the NHS was widely regarded as being the best health system in the world.

I remain of the belief that this was so because we as Britons cared about the NHS, regarded it as being our NHS, took an active interest in informing themselves about the health system and, importantly, assumed a wider social responsibility for protecting it.

From an early age we were taught to raise our voices if we had any concerns (we are not called 'Whinging Poms' for nothing), and I remain of the belief this is why Britain had one of the best health systems in the world. Collectively we would raise our voices and say something if we thought something was wrong with any aspect of the NHS, and would hold people to account for what they did or failed to do within our health system.

So my advice to you is this: if you want to have one of the best health systems in the world, you have to take an active interest in it. You have to assume a social responsibility for it and you must play your part in protecting it.

This may mean doing the most simple of things such as asking for the soap dispenser to be refilled when it is empty, rather than simply rubbing your hands together under the running tap, to doing such things as lobbying your local minister to reinstate the local bus service to the hospital, calling on your local hospitals to adequately staff wards, or acting to prevent your local public hospitals from being privatised.

Remember, this is YOUR health system. You are the eyes and ears of the health system, and you are often the only ones who see things as they really are. This is often long after the nurses and doctors have stopped seeing or have simply given up trying to change things.

Be silent, and I promise you that health authorities and successive governments will decide your public health system is too expensive to maintain and they will arbitrarily dismantle it, pay award by pay award, staff member by staff member, bed by bed and hospital by hospital until you barely have a public health system left. And if you think I am being unnecessarily alarmist, then consider these Federal Government treasury forward estimates for the 7 year period from 2017 to 2024. It is estimated that the Federal Government will reduce health spending by 57 billion dollars.

Questioning, challenging and changing detrimental cultural practices

Some of you have been raised in cultures or within households where as children you learnt it was acceptable to spit and empty your nostrils directly onto the street and in communal settings.

Some of you have not traditionally had access to adequate supplies of clean water, and so you have not learnt to wash your hands before and after meals, and before food preparation.

Still others of you have found it acceptable to let others breast-feed your children, have traditionally touched the bodies of those who have died of infectious diseases, or have let untrained or unqualified people carry out surgical procedures on your children.

This has to stop.

If we are to avoid the spread of communicable infections and adverse health outcomes, everyone must play their part in preventing these things from happening in the future. This involves learning from reputable sources such as your GP or from the health department in your local area about how to do this, or how to prevent this from happening.

Participating in health research

One of the most difficult, costly, and time-consuming aspects of doing health research is finding research participants. These include people who have the disease or illness they wish to research, or people of comparable age and backgrounds who can act as controls for the research.

I would strongly urge you become involved by registering as research volunteers and participating in research studies. You can do this by either contacting your nearest research hospital or registering online as a research volunteer. I am currently involved with 'Register4' and the Sax Institute's longitudinal '45 and Up' study. Information about this register and research study can be found at www.register4.org.au and www.saxinstritute.org.au. Visit these websites to see how these types of registers and studies work, and how you can volunteer to help further research in the future.

While you might not personally directly benefit from such research studies, they will almost certainly benefit others. These people could be your children or extended kin in the future. Consider this as being one of your lasting legacies.

Engage in benevolent gestures

While most of us are familiar with the need for people to become blood or organ donors, there are other ways you can assist individual patients, and advancements in medicine and forensic science generally. These include:

- Become a bone marrow donor. For more information: www.abmdr.org.au

- Donate your baby's cord blood globally to the National Cord Blood Collection and Banking Network. For more information: www.abmdr.org.au

- Donate your body to the 'Body Farm'. For more information, contact Professor Shari Forbes at the University of Technology, Sydney (UTS). Her current email address is: shari.forbes@uts.edu.au

- Donate your body or organs to medical science such as the Brain Donor program in Sydney University. For

more information:
www.abc.net.au/science/articles/204/05/27/2857045.htm

Investing in health research and innovations

Apart from participating in health research as a research volunteer or becoming a donor, you might want to also consider investing in health research and in health innovations if you are in a financial position to do so.

Many health research projects being run though our universities and research hospitals require your financial backing, and there are plenty of crowd sourcing opportunities to invest in health innovations. Some of these such as Cochlear have provided excellent returns for their investors since listing on the stock market. Again, consider this as being one of your lasting legacies and one which may benefit you or one of your family members in the future.

Author's note

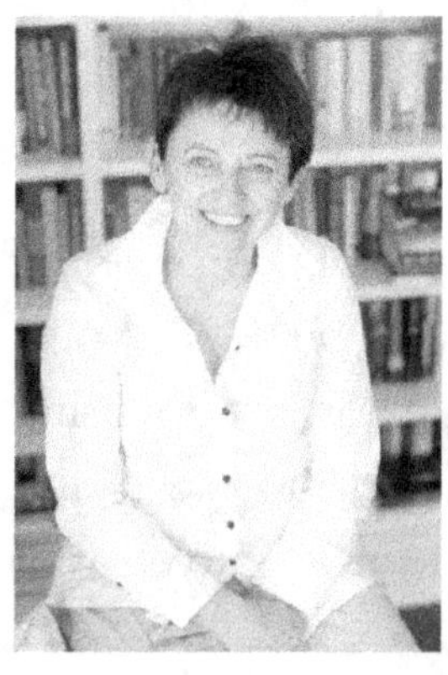

As you can imagine, I might face criticism from some quarters when this book is published. To my detractors and critics I would say but one thing: you have to say it how it is and how you find it. It is no good sugar-coating a person's expectation of what the health system is and can be when this does not adhere to reality.

As a highly experienced registered nurse and person in this wider community, I have a legal, moral and ethical responsibility to protect patients. This is what I am endeavouring to do with this book. I am trying to do this by telling people how it is, and where and how things can go wrong for them as patients. Importantly I am advising them how they can potentially protect themselves and others as patients in the future.

Some of you will say that I am politicising health and needlessly frightening people, and that I am putting people off from seeking treatment as a patient. To you I say this: Our health system has been politicised and some people are already too frightened to seek treatment as patients. In my experience as a community nurse, I know some people have been deeply traumatised by what they have personally experienced or have witnessed happening to others in hospital. People have openly expressed a wish to die at home rather than to go into hospital.

Far from frightening them still further, I anticipate this book will serve to empower them by giving them the knowledge and confidence with which they can protect themselves. This knowledge will enable them to act and raise their concerns and will provide them with the justification and legitimacy for doing so.

Some of you will also criticise me for using technical language and will say I am being elitist by only appealing to a certain percentage of the population who can read this book. To you I say this: if someone is going to complain, or act to bring awareness to things they now know are wrong in the health system, they are going to find themselves in an adversarial position at times.

If they are to be listened to and taken seriously and not simply dismissed or ignored, they are going to have to know, or at least be familiar with the technical language of those who would make them their foes. And whilst some people will have difficulty with this book, I anticipate that some of their friends, colleagues, supporters and children will not.

In saying this, however, I would like to hear from you if you have any criticisms about what I have written and I will consider your criticism. With this in mind my email address for any criticisms of this book is makeacontribution@gmail.com. Please put 'Criticism' in the subject section of the email.

I would also like to hear from those people who value and have been helped by the book, and from professional colleagues who think of something else I should have included. I am always happy to hear from you. Regard this as being a collegial effort to benefit and to improve the life of patients in the future. You can use the same email for any contributions you wish to make. Simply write 'Suggestion' in the subject section of the email.

Contributions will be credited to those who make them.

Finally, many of you as my peers and colleagues have already praised me for writing this book, and have gone as far as to say it has been long overdue and should have been written sooner. Some of you have asked to read it when it is published. To you I say: "thanks for your support and interest", and I would wish you to know that I do so with deep gratitude and heartfelt thanks.

Kate Ryder
Sydney, Australia, 2015